HEALTH CARE ISSUES, COSTS AND ACCESS

END-OF-LIFE CARE

ETHICAL ISSUES, PRACTICES AND CHALLENGES

Health Care Issues, Costs and Access

Additional books in this series can be found on Nova's website under the Series tab.

Additional e-books in this series can be found on Nova's website under the e-book tab.

HEALTH CARE ISSUES, COSTS AND ACCESS

END-OF-LIFE CARE

ETHICAL ISSUES, PRACTICES AND CHALLENGES

MARIA ROSSI
AND
LUIZ ORTIZ
EDITORS

nova publishers
New York

For permission to use material from this book please contact us:
Telephone 631-231-7269; Fax 631-231-8175
Web Site: http://www.novapublishers.com

Additional color graphics may be available in the e-book version of this book.

Library of Congress Cataloging-in-Publication Data

Library of Congress Control Number: 2013944379

ISBN: 978-1-62808-555-6

Published by Nova Science Publishers, Inc. † New York

CONTENTS

PREFACE

Human death is a mystery. Although scientists have identified the criteria, states, and signs of biological death, undoubtedly the issues of dying and death have a wider meaning. In this book, the authors present current research in the study of the ethical issues, practices and challenges of end-of-life care. Topics discussed include the challenges in heart failure and end-of-life care; a spiritual perspective of end-of-life experiences; a veterinary oncologist's interprofessional crossover perspective of euthanasia for terminal patients; diabetes and end-of-life care; helping families to cope after the death of a loved one; multidimensional aspects of nursing care for dying patients; spirituality at the end-of-life; challenges of promoting end-of-life care in residential care homes in Hong Kong; and the current situation and challenges of home end-of-life care for the elderly in Japan.

Chapter 1 – Significant, irreversible deterioration in cardiac function and output is a key marker of impending mortality and requires careful end of life care planning. There are currently 1 million patients diagnosed with heart failure in the United Kingdom and 6 million in the United States and many more patients have undiagnosed heart failure. A leading cause of hospitalisation, heart failure patients have multiple end of life needs including symptom control, psychological, social and spiritual support, akin to terminal cancer patients, yet the provision of services and support facilities are far less developed and utilised. Patients and their care givers, including clinicians are also not as well informed about the condition and its prognosis. UK guidelines have highlighted the necessity for improved end of life discussions and unmet palliative needs in heart failure, and focus on community based approaches to end of life planning involving an appointed professional coordinating care with specialist medical and palliative support to increase service provision. Models have shown this has enabled more patients to die at home with only few requiring specialist input. Despite acknowledging the need for early integration of services, this is still poorly executed in the majority of cases. Barriers to effective and timely end of life planning in heart failure include lack of physician training, patient misconception of what is involved and significantly, the difficulty in accurate prognostication and when to initiate such discussions. Inpatient mortality from heart failure can be predicted using scoring methods such as the widely validated 'Get With The Guidelines - Heart Failure' risk score. Such scores can help identify those patients for full medical salvage versus palliation alone and can trigger timely end of life discussions. Although they could still be improved with the addition of biomarker parameters, routine use of scores on admission would help facilitate decision making between patients, care givers and medical professionals. The scores could trigger the involvement of appropriate support services and improve overall patient experience and reduce hospital admissions or length of inpatient stay. If applied wisely in the community to patients with no further therapeutic options, they may enable patients to die with dignity in an environment of their choice, such as their home or hospice without the need for admission, where the focus is on recovery and not palliation. An additional component in heart failure patients is the use of implantable cardiac defibrillators, cardiac resynchronisation therapy and left ventricular assist devices. The ethics of timing of withdrawing or deactivating these therapies has been the focus of much work, helping patients and relatives and clinicians to recognise when these measures are appropriate. All of these complexities make heart failure perhaps the most challenging discipline for end of life planning. Considerable work is therefore needed in raising the profile, providing the tools and generating the evidence base for best management to address these issues. This chapter will discuss these challenges and provide multiple perspectives and some solutions but the field requires further development and additional improvement.

Chapter 2 – Spiritual awareness is an important part of care for the dying. the authors' research with a palliative care team, and with the carers in hospices and a nursing home, has confirmed that end-of-life experiences, which occur in the last few days of life have spiritual implications for the dying and their families, and are not uncommon. These experiences include visions by the dying, usually of dead relatives, deathbed 'coincidences', in which someone emotionally close to a dying person reports being 'visited' by them at the time of their death, and the feeling of going into and out of another reality. Carers of the dying also report that at the moment of death they may see something leaving the body or light surrounding it. Carers also report the desire which the dying often show for reconciliation with their life and, importantly other family members. Nearly all the reports (85%) suggested that these experiences are profoundly comforting both to the dying themselves, and to any family members who witness the phenomena. The study has clear implications for theories about the continuation of consciousness after death. New studies on after-death experiences during cardiac arrest, in which patients report seeing the resuscitation process, suggest that the authors' current model of brain function may need to be expanded. One interpretation of the data is that it may point to a continuation of consciousness.

Chapter 3 – Diabetes is the most significant chronic disease and the global prevalence is increasing. Diabetes is associated with debilitating long term complications and other comorbidities that cause high rates of morbidity and mortality. Keeping blood glucose and other metabolic parameters within an acceptable, personalised range is important to comfort and quality of life but can be challenging, especially during end-of-life care. Guidelines can help clinicians make appropriate care decisions; however, there is little research about what constitutes best practice diabetes care at the end-of-life: existing recommendations and guidelines blend the best available evidence with consensus opinion. In addition, there are important ethical and methodological considerations concerning research involving vulnerable people at the end-of-life. Chapter 3 describes the ethical and methodological issues that needed to be considered when developing guidelines for managing diabetes at the end-of-life and the contribution interviews with dying people and their family carers made to developing a guiding philosophy and to person-centred guidelines.

Chapter 4 – The End-of-Life Care requires a global and holistic approach to provide an excellent care, meeting the needs of both, the person who is dying and their relatives. In this sense, it is important to recognize that the family, including close friends and carers, has a vital role during this process. They need to be closely involved in their loved one care as well as they have their own needs, which are not only present before and during death but also after the person's death. Good end of life care does not stop at the point of death, and the proper emotional support is required by family members and friends to cope with their loss. After the loss of a loved person, -one of the most stressful and painful events that people experience in their lives-, bereavement appears as a natural response. Most of people come to terms with this universal experience without requiring specialized psychotherapy. However, for a significant minority of bereaved people who struggle deeply and for a prolonged period of time, grief is complicated. In those circumstances we would be talking about complicated grief or prolonged grief disorder. The aim of this chapter is to revise the main issues related to grief and bereavement, including the definition of these terms, stages and tasks of grief, the description of the different types of grief reactions, complicated grief and treatments for helping bereaved people.

Chapter 5 – Human death is a mystery. Although scientists have identified the criteria, states, and signs of biological death, undoubtedly the issues of dying and death have a wider meaning. In this paper the authors would like to emphasize the multidimensional character of the process of dying and nursing care offered during this period. This type of care is tightly associated with various ethical problems and dilemmas. This results from subjectively assessed health-related quality of life, among others. The dilemmas pertain to patient's expectations and decisions made by his/her loved ones or the members of therapeutic team. Starting another regimen of anticancer treatment and reducing the dose of pain medications in order to avoid addiction, the patient meets the expectations of his/her loved ones; frequently these expectations represent unmitigated fight for life. Is such attitude always beneficial for the patient? The lack of universal solutions is reflected by various controversies pertaining both to the crucial decisions and to the selection of the methods and way of care. Nursing care is related to all dimensions of human being: biological, psychological, social, spiritual, and cultural ones. The care should be offered both to the dying patient and to his/her loved ones. Esteem, friendliness, empathy, openness, as well as the ability and accuracy of responding to somatic suffering seem to be both the source of support and the sign of care for a patient and his/her family. Professional career of a nurse comprises various stages associated with realizing her abilities with regards to life, dying, and death. The professionalism of a nurse can be manifested by her creative presence, care, assistance, and consolation; however, it is not always possible to get rid of the feeling of helplessness, lack of acceptance to passing away, and other strong emotions in view of patient's death. During this study the authors talked to terminally-ill patients of a hospice. This research confirmed that every human being dies differently. The authors have been surprised by various attitudes to death, as well as by different expectations toward accompanying persons. Not only each dying person is different as an individual, also his/her mood and mental status change rapidly and sometimes unexpectedly. Also this finding emphasizes the importance and difficulties associated with care for terminally-ill patients. The above mentioned observations suggest that despite nurses' experience in accompanying dying individuals, one should not create any universal model of care for this group of patients.

Chapter 6 – Facing death and the pain of the separation and the different losses is hard to bear for all those concerned. An important part of patient's discomfort does not come directly from the disease but from its subjective experience. At this regard, physical or biological needs should be addressed, as well as social, emotional and spiritual ones. Currently, it is recognized that spiritual factors may play an important role in the patient's serenity and suffering. For this reason this group of needs would have a great value, especially in the context of the end-of-life, where people cope with an array of difficulties and stressors, such as pain, feelings of uncertainty, and many changes at different levels because of the progression and irreversibility of the illness. But what do we understand by spiritual needs? To define the concept of spirituality is not an easy task. Despite the fact that traditionally both terms, spirituality and religion, were practically inseparable, it is important not to confuse them. Spirituality is broader than religion, and an individual can be spiritual without being religious. This and other issues related to the spirituality at the end-of-life, such as the search for personal and psychological meaning, will be addressed in the present chapter.

Chapter 7 – Growing attention is being paid to the healthcare needs of older people who live with advanced diseases or disabilities. Studies have shown that frail older people share similar concerns and needs as patients who have terminal diseases. End-of-life care should therefore be extended to older people who are experiencing a progressive worsening of their health and functional ability. In Hong Kong, older people living in residential care homes are relatively frailer because moving to a long-term care setting is usually the last resort when their substantial care needs cannot be met at home. Hence, a residential care home is an optimal place for promoting end-of-life care. However, end-of-life care has yet to be systematically integrated into the care practice in this setting. This chapter will discuss three major challenges in promoting end-of-life care in residential care homes for older people: (1) whether Chinese older people are willing to openly talk about issues of death and dying; (2) whether family members and healthcare providers are willing to support end-of-life care provision; and (3) whether end-of-life care development is facilitated in the community.

Expert Commentary – This discussion is an expert commentary on why and how society seems to maintain a dual ethic on standards for quality of life at the end-of-life between animal vs. human patients. Due to the cherished value of the human-animal bond in society, veterinary medical practitioners adopted the pediatrician model. The unique difference between a small animal practitioner's vs. a pediatrician's end-of-life approach is that their companion animal patients are considered geriatric babies! The author is a practicing veterinary oncologist with 40 plus years of experience serving clients and their animal cancer patients with Pawspice, a practice which simultaneously embraces both palliative and standard care. When quality of life (QoL) declines to the point where the patient can no longer enjoy life, clients are compassionately counseled to consider the gift of humane euthanasia for their beloved pets. When pet owners fail to recognize the relentless suffering and frustration of their dying companion animals, the attending veterinary medical staff endures distress which may result in a nagging moral stress that makes them more prone to compassion fatigue. Veterinarians serve society as healers. They have the oath and responsibility of compassionately preventing suffering in their patients. This includes preventing the misery and anguish of being forced to endure a prolonged or bad death. Human longing for euthanasia is especially fulminate when the body is in relentless decline yet being kept in suspension to scientifically defy death. This is accomplished very well via modern medicine and life supportive care in ICU's and skilled nursing homes. The science ideology that death can and should be defeated, no matter the cost, is standard of practice for a large majority of physicians. This unique thinking is very American. It is encouraged by the innovative for-profit medical marketplace which has not yet defeated the inevitability of death. Physician detachment from death is unsustainable and imposes great emotional stress on patients and their families and a foreboding expense on the health care system for baby boomers.

Short Communication – Although a number of elderly people are opting to spend their last few years of life at home, elderly home end-of-life care has not yet gained popularity in Japan. In this short communication paper, the authors describe the current situation, and outline the challenges of home end-of-life care for the elderly in Japan using the KJ method as qualitative research tool.

In: End-of-Life Care
Editors: Maria Rossi and Luiz Ortiz
ISBN: 978-1-62808-555-6

Chapter 1

END-OF-LIFE CARE: ETHICAL ISSUES, PRACTICES AND CHALLENGES IN HEART FAILURE

Anna Steel and Ameet Bakhai*

Department of Cardiology, Barnet & Chase Farm Hospitals NHS Trust, Wellhouse Lane, Barnet, Herts, UK

ABSTRACT

Significant, irreversible deterioration in cardiac function and output is a key marker of impending mortality and requires careful end of life care planning. There are currently 1 million patients diagnosed with heart failure in the United Kingdom and 6 million in the United States and many more patients have undiagnosed heart failure. A leading cause of hospitalisation, heart failure patients have multiple end of life needs including symptom control, psychological, social and spiritual support, akin to terminal cancer patients, yet the provision of services and support facilities are far less developed and utilised. Patients and their care givers, including clinicians are also not as well informed about the condition and its prognosis. UK guidelines have highlighted the necessity for improved end of life discussions and unmet palliative needs in heart failure, and focus on community based approaches to end of life planning involving an appointed professional coordinating care with specialist medical and

* Corresponding author: Dr Ameet Bakhai, Department of Cardiology, Barnet Hospital, Wellhouse Lane, Barnet, Herts, EN5 3DJ, Email: abakhai@nhs.net.

palliative support to increase service provision. Models have shown this has enabled more patients to die at home with only few requiring specialist input. Despite acknowledging the need for early integration of services, this is still poorly executed in the majority of cases. Barriers to effective and timely end of life planning in heart failure include lack of physician training, patient misconception of what is involved and significantly, the difficulty in accurate prognostication and when to initiate such discussions. Inpatient mortality from heart failure can be predicted using scoring methods such as the widely validated 'Get With The Guidelines - Heart Failure' risk score. Such scores can help identify those patients for full medical salvage versus palliation alone and can trigger timely end of life discussions. Although they could still be improved with the addition of biomarker parameters, routine use of scores on admission would help facilitate decision making between patients, care givers and medical professionals. The scores could trigger the involvement of appropriate support services and improve overall patient experience and reduce hospital admissions or length of inpatient stay. If applied wisely in the community to patients with no further therapeutic options, they may enable patients to die with dignity in an environment of their choice, such as their home or hospice without the need for admission, where the focus is on recovery and not palliation. An additional component in heart failure patients is the use of implantable cardiac defibrillators, cardiac resynchronisation therapy and left ventricular assist devices. The ethics of timing of withdrawing or deactivating these therapies has been the focus of much work, helping patients and relatives and clinicians to recognise when these measures are appropriate. All of these complexities make heart failure perhaps the most challenging discipline for end of life planning. Considerable work is therefore needed in raising the profile, providing the tools and generating the evidence base for best management to address these issues. This chapter will discuss these challenges and provide multiple perspectives and some solutions but the field requires further development and additional improvement.

The Burden of Heart Failure

Heart failure is one of the leading causes of death in the western world [1]. In our setting of the United Kingdom (UK) with a population of 63 million, it is estimated that around one million citizens are living with heart failure [2] with a direct resource use of £600 million to the National Health Service per annum [3]. The risk of developing heart failure is greater as the population ages, with the annual incidence being over four times higher in those aged 85 and over, compared to those aged 65 and over. [4]. Heart failure is the leading cause of hospitalisation, involved directly or indirectly, for one in every five admissions in those aged 65 and over, with increasing numbers of admissions as the disease progresses [5]. The REMATCH (Randomised Evaluation of Mechanical Assistance for the Treatment of Congestive Heart Failure) trial showed that in the last two years of life, patients with heart failure spent on average 82.8 days in hospital, which increased to one in every four days in the final six months of life [6]. Improving end of life care for patients with heart failure has therefore been identified as a national priority in the UK [7]. Despite this priority, new European Society of Cardiology guidance in heart failure released in 2012 stated that end of life care in heart failure was a recognised area with a gap in the evidence base and gave little direction on ideal management.

In addition to poor prognosis of the disease, there is considerable reduction in the quality of life of patients with heart failure, due to disabling symptoms and numerous unmet psychological, social and spiritual needs [8,9]. These symptoms are not only present prior to a diagnosis but for many patients the symptoms remain despite treatment and then worsen after disease progression beyond the benefits of therapy. Fatigue, breathlessness, fluid retention (oedema) and sleep disturbance are most commonly seen symptoms in end stage disease and prior to diagnosis. Factors associated with increased symptoms include being female, having two or more other co-morbidities and concomitant depression [10,11]. The survival rate for heart failure is worse than for many cancers, with similar rates of one year mortality at 38% [12] increasing to 60% within five years [13]. Many of the end stage symptoms overlap with those commonly found in cancer patients such as pain, fatigue, loss of independence, difficulty in walking, anxiety, lack of confidence and depression. *Both cancer and heart failure sufferers also have significant psychological burdens yet far fewer heart failure patients receive social, functional or psychological support [14].*

In general, cancer patients are better informed about their condition than heart failure patients, with greater awareness of their prognosis, involvement in decision making and better access to social, health and financial support services. In contrast, heart failure patients were frustrated, more socially isolated and stressed due to managing a complex condition and underutilised various care services available to them. Heart failure patients often did not understand the terminal nature of their disease, had not entered any end of life discussions and had less opportunity to die at home [15]. Despite the disease burden being similar in both conditions, care services appear to be prioritised based on diagnosis rather than individual need, resulting in care that is not patient centred and inequitable.

One additional frustration is that the term heart failure is the most internationally recognised phrase to label this condition, despite the fact that the heart has failed while the individual is alive. A more accurate term would be cardiac output impairment (either compensated or decompensated). In contrast, gene replication failure is known as cancer, coronary circulation failure as a heart attack, brain failure as stroke or dementia, pancreas failure as diabetes mellitus, kidney failure as chronic kidney disease or acute kidney injury and failure to conceive as infertility. Heart failure once given as a diagnosis, results in an uphill psychological battle for patients, carers and the clinicians dealing with these individuals.

National Guidelines and Policy Matters in End of Life Care in Heart Failure – The United Kingdom Example

The UK is blessed with a single, majority health care provider (National Health Service). This allows us to examine how the focus of care has evolved in the last decade through easy to retrieve policy and guidance documents all readily available in the public domain, providing us with an insightful timeline on end of life care in heart failure. Palliative care need of heart failure patients were first documented as a major issue in NHS policy in 2000 [16] and then highlighted in the national guidelines on heart failure management in 2003, with emphasis on the need for end of life care planning [17]. In 2004 the national guidelines for supportive and palliative care for advanced heart failure [18] were based mostly on cancer guidelines and discussed the need for improved communication skills for clinicians diagnosing the condition. Moving further to focus on the patient, the NHS 'End of life care pathway' in 2008 highlighted the need for more open end of life discussions between clinicians and patients [19]. The UK End-of-Life Care Strategy then identified the assessment of patient need as a marker of quality of care [20].

An unusual situation in heart failure is that clinicians and manufacturers have focused on reducing the risk of sudden death in heart failure by implanting specialised cardiac pacemakers, with the ability to monitor for and intervene on fatal rhythm disturbances with internal electric shocks, known as implantable cardiac defibrillators. As more patients are given such expensive and complex devices, in addition to symptom relief, recent cardiology guidelines have focused on policies related to the withdrawal of the defibrillation therapy in the final stages of heart failure [21,22]. This does not involve stopping the pacing function of these devices to keep the heart attempting to pump, only the ability to prevent the fatal rhythm disturbances. This subject has highlighted how essential good communication has been around the act of reprogramming devices, which has sometimes been misperceived by patients and relatives as a terminal act in itself, although the reality is far from this as only the defibrillation function is removed and not the pacing function. Many patients and carers have commented that such communication was also not provided prior to device implantation, which shows how expensive, complex therapies are being prescribed without patients and carers feeling they have been fully informed or engaged, despite consenting procedures.

The National Institute for Health and Care Excellence (NICE) which provides comprehensive, evidence based guidelines to secure high quality care in the NHS, has stated in the 2010 guidelines that 'there is substantive evidence for considerable, unmet, palliative needs of patients with heart failure' and 'areas of need include symptom control, psychological and social support, planning for the future and end of life care'. *The guidelines include the need for honest and accurate information to be tailored to individual patients, good communication and involvement of patients, carers and relatives in the management and discussion of prognosis [18].*

Another major national initiative in the UK, known as the National Service Framework for coronary heart disease, an initiative to reduce premature mortality due to coronary disease, also recognises the need for palliative care for heart failure patients. It advocates structured care through use of a heart disease register and treatment protocols shared across local care networks (including primary care in the community with secondary and tertiary care from general and specialist hospitals). Mentioned deliberately in the guidance are effective discharge planning after hospital admission and referral to social and community chronic disease services and also more recently an adoption of the World Health Organisation (WHO) palliative care approach in end-stage disease [17]. The department of health subsequently advocated the provision of palliative and end of life care in the last year of life regardless of diagnosis [19].

The UK experience teaches us, that it has taken over 12 years in a developed country to progress from identifying an unmet need to improve end of life communication to accepting the psychosocial needs of heart failure patients. Yet despite the growing acknowledgement of the need for integrated palliative care services, there has to date, not been sufficient investigation into appropriate models of care and little published guidance on how to provide these services in the context of heart failure specifically. Much work has yet to be done to emulate the support provided to cancer patients. Why this gap exists is multifactorial, including factors such as limitations in physician training, patients not voicing concerns and needs, unpredictable nature of the disease progression, availability of effective therapies and so on, but some key issues are worth discussing more fully.

End of Life Discussions and Early Integration of Palliative Care Services

End of life planning or "preparedness planning" is important for heart failure patients to allow discussion and planning for different modes of death and the most appropriate location of care for patients during the terminal phase of their disease. These discussions, to be led by the physician in charge, facilitate support for family and equally important, the caregivers in the event of death and improved understanding of the disease process and overall quality of life [23]. Advanced directives from the patients are also consistently underutilised in heart failure and such discussions allow us to visit these options. Both older and more recent studies have shown this perpetuating trend on advance directives [24] with one study highlighting that only 24% of patients knew what advanced directives were, yet when it was explained to them 80% wanted to discuss the concept with a clinician [25]. Advanced directives should be discussed soon after diagnosis of heart failure and are particularly useful when deciding on the implantation or deactivation of devices such as implantable cardiac defibrillator or left ventricular assist devices, which support the pumping function of the heart. A patient's goals and values should be ascertained to support patient autonomy and enable the most appropriate decisions to be made for that individual. For example, some patients prefer symptom control over survival [26] whilst others hold polar opinions regarding quality of life versus longevity [27]. It is also important to discuss resuscitation preferences in the context of a patient's beliefs and goals. These discussions should also begin early and the important points of the discussion revisited at timely intervals to ensure that the patient's on-going needs are met such as additional co-morbidities or changes in personal outlook.

One reason that heart failure management has been fragmented is that traditionally cardiologists and general physicians diagnosing patients with heart failure have not had personal training in end of care issues, nor do they enlist the care of palliative care specialists early [28]. These clinicians are often so engaged with the clinical therapeutic decisions to be made that they do not then focus on the psychosocial aspects. Sometimes this is because there is no structured sequence of discussions around heart failure and therefore inadequate time and resources dedicated to all areas of need. Meeting these additional needs to encourage delivery of information to patients and care-givers, not only improves overall management but also may reduce unplanned hospitalisation rates [29,30]. Addressing symptoms such as depression will also reduce symptom burden and unplanned hospital admissions [11].

Barriers to End of Life Discussions

Physician Factors

As discussed, doctors often face barriers to having end of life discussions and involving palliative care services with heart failure patients. There are several reasons for this to explore further. The first concern is about giving bad news too soon or saying the wrong thing at a stage when patient physician relationship is still developing, with the risk that patient may give up the 'fight for life' [31]. Cardiologists and cardiac nurses are often unfamiliar with the principles and approaches of palliative care [32] and feel they do not have the necessary skills to manage these [33] due to *a lack of lack of expertise in palliative care or formal training [28]*. Although the WHO guidelines state that palliative intervention is applicable in early disease alongside more commonly used treatment options [34], few clinicians are able to determine at the early stage which patients have pre-terminal heart failure and which patients are salvageable as the number of variables affecting the outcome are so numerous. Often when heart failure is diagnosed, there are numerous investigations into cause and severity that are yet to be completed and then management options are wide ranging from medications, revascularisation and specialised pacemakers to transplantation and ventricular assist devices. So the early stage of the disease is often focused on aetiology, search for reversible factors and prognosis. These concepts alone are so involving in discussions with complex terms and tests that there is often less time to focus on end stage discussions for the same clinician. Indeed mixing discussions on what can be repaired with planning for the end stage is a skill few clinicians manage without confusing the patient and caregivers.

Patient Factors

Patients also have barriers to accepting palliative care due to the stigma and misconception of the role of palliative care specialists. Patients and relatives often believe that meeting palliative care specialists implies that death is imminent and that the cardiologist have exhausted their consideration of treatment options. They do not recognise that the palliative care team provide insight, reassurance, respite care and better symptom control both during the management stage and at the end stage of heart failure care. Poor patient understanding of prognosis also acts as a barrier to open end of life care planning. For example, in one study, while most patients had planned their funeral, they had not discussed their preferred place of death with their doctor [35], illustrating a disparity between doctor-patient discussions and a patient's perspective on their lifespan. *Clinicians and patients often wait for each other to bring up end of life conversations which frequently results in no discussion at all [36].* In cancer management, discussion about end of life issues has resulted in fewer invasive interventions and improved quality of life in the terminal stages of disease for patients. The information given did not depress or scare patients any more than patients who had not engaged in such discussions [37]. Empowering relatives with information also impacts positively on their psychological recovery after patient death.

Disease Factors

With heart failure, one of the major difficulties in allocating palliative care services appropriately is due to the variable presentation stages of congestive cardiac failure. Mortality rates among heart failure patients range widely, between 5 -75% in the first year, and death can be sudden due to fatal cardiac rhythm disorders despite oral medications or slower and more progressive as a result of pump failure and progressive loss of cardiac output. This divergent mode of death makes prediction difficult [38] and many doctors often see themselves as poor prognosticators and have suggested that nurses, carers and even the patients are more realistic predictors [31]. *In contrast to the unpredictable demise in heart failure, cancer patients enjoy a relatively high functional level prior to a rapid, progressive decline that prompts the timely intervention of palliative care.*

Thus several aspects of heart failure require tackling from physician training needs to patient insight into the involvement of palliative care team, from accurate prognosis prediction tools to appropriate involvement of non-clinical carers and relatives.

PREDICTION OF PROGNOSIS IN HEART FAILURE

To reduce the prognostic uncertainty in heart failure, various models have been formulated to aid prediction of death. The Seattle Heart Failure Model (SHFM) is one of the most widely validated predictive tools used in the out-patient setting in heart failure [38]. The 'Get With The Guidelines' Heart Failure (GWTG-HF) risk score is a validated predictive model and is specific for in-patient mortality. It uses readily available clinical data that enables prediction of mortality at initial presentation after hospital admission [39]. The tool has been widely validated across almost 200 US hospitals including over 39,500 patients with diverse demographic characteristics and co-morbidities. Other models include the ADHERE score and the OPTIMIZE-HF score. These other models however use very few variables or are less widely validated [38,40]. The GWTG-HF risk score uses seven parameters and can be easily calculated at the bedside, making it highly accessible for use by clinicians [39]. Further investigation is still required to determine the accuracy of the prognostic information and whether the score can be utilised prospectively in order to make difficult management decisions.

Recently, further studies suggest that the addition of a biomarker parameter can further improve the accuracy of HF mortality prediction scores such as the SHFM [41]. Further investigation has found that assessing multiple biomarkers with clinical parameters provides a composite risk factor score that is superior to biomarkers used in isolation [42]. Further investigation is needed to more fully assess the value of including biomarkers such as B-naturetic peptide (BNP) and troponin to both in-patient and out-patient scoring systems. These biomarkers are sensitive measures of cardiac myocyte strain and damage and in the case of BNP have become more widely available and used, only in the last 5 years. Additional factors such as cardiac imaging parameters of atrial stretch, presence of myocardial and in particular intraventricular septal fibrosis, nutritional status, albumin level, mobility and the presence of pulmonary oedema also need to be integrated into scoring systems as each of these have prognostic value in smaller detailed studies but have not all been evaluated simultaneously in larger studies.

Linking Prediction with Palliative and Specialist Input

The use of clinical triggers for involvement of palliative services has been discussed by various guideline groups as one solution to managing end of life issues here. The Heart Failure Association of the European Society of Cardiology suggested such involvement be considered for any of the following [43]:

- multiple episodes of decompensation within a duration of six months despite optimal therapy,
- malignant rhythm disorders,
- requirement of intravenous treatment with inotropes to support cardiac output,
- a chronic poor quality of life,
- (NHYA class IV) symptoms of breathlessness at rest
- or the presence of cardiac cachexia.

A simpler approach from the Gold Standards Framework suggests using more pragmatic criteria such as asking the patient if they agreed with the statement: 'death in the next 12 months would not be a surprise' [44]. Methods such as these are however open to subjective interpretation, such as assessing the quality of life or in what context the patient is asked the question about their own potential mortality. Similarly confusing is that the methods may be identifying people who could have greater benefit from complex salvage strategies such as pacemakers or ventricular assist devices, rather than predict who will die despite such therapies. Such therapies themselves carry a small risk and therefore these therapies have a lower benefit to risk ratio in less ill patients.

Further insights from the large UK national audit of 37,076 records of patients (National Heart Failure Audit 2012 report) admitted overnight, showed that much of heart failure patient admissions still resides in the care of general physicians, with 52% of patients being dealt with fully on non-cardiology wards during admission [45]. Many clinicians feel cardiology could not cope with caring for all heart failure related admissions, given a lack of dedicated manpower. This has led to the delayed or deferred input during admission from specialists dedicated to heart failure, let alone palliative care. Thus an additional benefit of a mortality prediction score can help to trigger the involvement of specialist cardiology and palliative services, initiate discussion and coordination between different specialties and thus achieve a better outcome for the patient along the disease course. For example, if patients were reviewed by a specialist heart failure team then more up to date management could be delivered, such as rapid fluid removal for symptom control (diuresis or ultrafiltration) where appropriate. Prognostication is a useful guide when deciding on mode of treatment but it should not be the sole driver behind decisions on therapy. In our opinion, a holistic and multidisciplinary approach which engages patients and caregivers from early on in the disease course, frequently addressing patient needs, enables the best care from the patient perspective to be delivered. Specialist leaders who promote an integrated approach in management are still the exception in heart failure care.

As well as helping to trigger the involvement of different specialties and patient discussion, formal computed prognostication can help identify patients who should be considered for alternative placement for their care, other than hospital [46]. Admission to hospital for many patients at the end of the disease course is also inappropriate. Many such patients would benefit from the holistic care given in hospices or may be most comfortable at home. Identifying those with poor mortality prediction scores can help facilitate the patient dying with dignity in an appropriate environment of their choice, rather than a busy general ward where other patients are being admitted and discharged rapidly, with more physical than psychosocial needs.

Device Treatment for Advanced Heart Failure

Cardiac transplantation is the 'gold standard' for refractory heart failure, but with less than 5000 donor hearts available per year worldwide, chances of survival on a waiting list is low [47]. Many patients are also considered ineligible for transplantation due to their functional state, age or other co-morbidities, which would not allow them to tolerate the immunosuppression medications needed in conjunction with transplantation. As a result implantable devices such as left ventricular assist devices (LVADs), implantable cardiac defibrillators (ICDs) and cardiac resynchronization therapy (CRT) have become available treatments, where optimal medication therapy is insufficient, but at considerable expense. LVADs were traditionally used as a 'bridge to transplant' to help extend survival whilst the waiting list but they are now more commonly being used as 'destination therapy' (DT) to enable functional recovery with stabilization on optimal medication only. The REMATCH trial [6] and the Investigation of Non-Transplant Eligible Patients who are Inotrope Dependent (INTrEPID) trial [48] have both demonstrated significantly improved survival data and improvements in quality of life for patients with LVADs versus those treated with maximum medical therapy, albeit with large economic expenditures to achieve this.

Another device solution in heart failure is the Implantable Cardiac Defibrillator, which treat lethal cardiac rhythm disturbances through overdrive pacing or shocks as needed. Clinical trials have demonstrated increased survival in those with previous sudden cardiac death, weakened hearts (ejection fraction less than 30-35%) and symptoms of breathlessness with moderate exertion (New York Heart Association class II) or worse [49]. Due to multiple studies showing the mortality benefit of ICDs, they are now most commonly implanted for primary prevention in heart failure [50], although many economies cannot afford the expenditures involved with widespread use of such technologies. Implantation of such devices are relatively low at 2% for mortality and around 2-6% for infection and the design of these devices continue to improve with new delivery models being trialed with leads outside the heart, further minimizing risk [51,52].

Cardiac resynchronization devices (CRT) are pacemakers that synchronize contraction of the two ventricles, reducing any efficiency loss between the ventricles if they do not contract simultaneously. These improve quality and length of life in patients with marked symptoms and weakened hearts (ejection fraction less than 35%) and wide QRS complex (>120ms) on the ECG, suggestive of incoordination or dyssynchrony. The Cardiac Resynchronization-Heart Failure (CARE-HF) study demonstrated a 36% relative risk reduction in the composite endpoint of all-cause mortality, improved quality of life, NYHA class of symptoms or hospital admission rates[53]. Many patients considered for such devices however are often ineligible and there is a procedural failure rate in achieving synchronization due to lead placement issues or limited programming optimization of the device [54]. The benefits of these devices are however often transient in many patients and so the key is appropriate selection of patients, often improved by the use of echo or cardiac MRI to measure dyssynchrony. Newer CRT devices are now available with both pacing function and also ICD technology as denoted by the classification CRT-D (with defibrillation). Naturally as the devices become more complex, then battery life becomes an issue as does device size and the complexity of the device implantation.

Important Considerations with Device Implantation

Careful discussion is required between clinicians, patients and carers before implantation of any complex cardiac implantable device. The benefits, limitations and effects on quality of life and quality of death, need extensive explanation. End of life planning for patients with devices should be common practice and commence before implantation as a matter of informed consent and as ongoing discussions throughout disease progression. It is also important to assess the health and abilities of the patient's carer, especially in the case of LVADs. Most patients with advanced heart failure are over 65 and in cases where the spouse/partner is the main carer, the onus and skills required can be extensive such as prevention of infection, maintenance of the device, dressing changes with sterile technique. These issues need careful consideration when discussing the effects of device implantation on a patient's and a carer's life.

When discussing implantation of LVADs it is important to point out that although there is an overall survival benefit and increased quality of life, there are still significant rates of infection, bleeding and stroke [55]. Ongoing assessment of quality of life is essential in patients with LVADs to ensure optimal patient-centered outcomes. An important point to consider with the implantation of ICDs, is the "quality of death" that patients may experience. An otherwise relatively painless and short terminal cardiac rhythm event can be converted into a period of prolonged suffering with significant heart failure symptoms by an ICD given to the wrong patient and not reprogrammed at the right time. Patients may receive multiple shocks in their final minutes, which can be very distressing if witnessed by family and caregivers. CRT devices prevent one death and three admissions for every nine devices implanted, however one third of patients do not get any benefit from the device and in some cases symptoms worsen [51]. It is still difficult to ascertain which patients will benefit and better predictive tools are again required.

ICDs and CRTs have been shown to be cost-effective in developed economies where hospital admissions are expensive [56]. LVADs however are still not considered cost-effective under current US guidelines [57]. They do however confer a significant improvement compared to the older pulsatile flow devices. With the potential for device usage to grow, cost to society needs to be considered. The assessment of cost-effectiveness uses quality-adjusted life years (QALYs) to evaluate quality of life together with prolonged survival. The use of these factors to gauge the merit of a treatment has been widely criticized regarding their ethical worth [58]. Concerns include how to define the value of a life, if age should influence medical priority and should the obligation to save a life outweigh competing values [59]. Criteria for QALYs to be ethically justifiable have been proposed but are not universally accepted. They include, (1) quality of life can be accurately measured and used, (2) utilitarianism is acceptable, (3) equity and efficiency are compatible, (4) projections of community preferences can substitute for individual preferences, (5) the old have less "capacity of benefit" than the young, and (6) physicians will not use quality-adjusted life years as clinical maxims [60]. Society values the preservation and improvement of life [61] however it is important to respect financial constraints where the payer is the state as in the UK. In such a situation clinicians again are put in tricky situations as to when to adhere to guidelines and restrictions or focus on individual patient level goals. Yet again few clinicians are trained in such complex clinical and economic thinking and holding multiple perspectives.

Deactivation of Devices

In advanced heart failure, devices such as ICDs prevent sudden cardiac death but increase the odds of pump failure related death. In certain situations, it becomes necessary to deactivate the shock function of the ICD if potential burdens outweigh the benefits due to the symptoms of advanced heart failure or other co-morbid diseases such as terminal cancer present. Some patients simply reach a stage when they prefer a natural death and the longevity of life is no longer their goal. Deactivation however is not always straight forward. Many ICDs have both the capability of pacing the heart as well as delivering shocks. For patients who develop slow heart rates at the end of life, the pacing feature of an ICD can relieve some of the symptoms such as fatigue and light-headedness. 'Overdrive pacing' is another feature which can terminate certain dysrhythmias without shocking. It is possible to disable certain functions of an ICD (e.g. the shock delivery function) and maintain these pacing elements [48]. It therefore becomes paramount that these situations are discussed as part of advanced care planning before the device is implanted. This would avoid such discussions taking place under the difficult circumstances of imminent death. Unfortunately, advanced planning and consideration of device deactivation is frequently missed [62,63]. In a recent study, most patients who had ICDs were unaware that they could be deactivated but 84% wanted to be able to discuss deactivation and many thought this should have been offered before implantation [64].

Deactivation of CRT devices pacing function will not provide any benefit in the end stages of life as it would primarily worsen heart failure symptoms [58] and therefore does not raise as many issues. LVADs offer good symptom control however they carry significant risks such as a stroke, sepsis or prolonged hospital admissions [65]. Thus advanced planning with deactivation discussion is necessary prior to implantation, before a potentially disabling event. The advance directive discussion should also include scenarios such as what to do if the LVAD fails and an emergency operation is required, or multi-organ failure occurs causing a 'futile' situation, or terminal malignancy develops. Discontinuation of LVADs is however difficult as it requires an operation. Many patients wish to die out of hospital but coordinating the technical expertise needed for removal of an LVAD and the provision of palliation at home or a hospice may be challenging. Deactivation of an LVAD is therefore usually a terminal event which raises contentious ethical arguments.

There is an important distinction between withholding and withdrawing treatment and the association with assisted suicide. There is little objection to withholding of treatment if the benefit does not outweigh the risks or the patient refuses the treatment. Broad consensus exists that it is justifiable to withdraw a life sustaining therapy which is no longer effective or causes more burden than benefit [66]. Withdrawal of external life support measures such as mechanical ventilation can be considered by some as 'passive assistance in dying'. The question with implantable devices is more complex as the device can be deemed as 'part of the patient' or an 'integral device' and thus discontinuation which hastens death can be likened to 'active assistance in dying' [67]. These different types of therapy can be labeled as 'replacement therapy' for an item that replaces a physiological function such as a transplanted organ or 'substitutive therapy' such as dialysis or assisted ventilation. There would be no question that removing or terminating a transplanted organ essential for life would constitute active killing. Withdrawing a substitutive therapy however is often essential and justifiable towards the end of life. It is questionable whether cardiac devices are replacement or substitutive, thus raising important discussion surrounding deactivation [68]. The argument is further complicated by the different device functions. Deactivation of the shock function of an ICD which is only recruited in the event of a life threatening dysrhythmia does not carry the same ethical problems as deactivation of a pacemaker in a patient who is pacemaker-dependent. Some argue that the patient's wishes should be the most important factor when making these ethical decisions and not a theoretical distinction [69] and deactivation should not differ to the refusal of other unwanted treatments [70]. Notably, from a legal perspective, no clinician has ever been found liable for wrongful death when following the wishes of a patient or surrogate, when withdrawing a life sustaining treatment [71].

The timing of device deactivation is also problematic. For ICDs, one study showed that for patients older than 84 and with renal impairment (glomerular filtration rate less than 39 ml/min), there was no survival benefit of a functional ICD [72], suggesting that these parameters could be used when considering if deactivation is appropriate. Others have developed models to guide advanced directive discussions with regard to deactivation. For instance, Petrucci et al. 2011 [73] provided a 10 point model to address ethical and psychosocial issues and advanced planning for patients receiving LVAD. As before prognostic scoring can trigger certain palliative measures towards the end of life including plans for discontinuation of devices. The only caveat to this is that the field of implantable devices continues to evolve and progress so that risks are decreasing and with increased targeting to the right patient at the right time, benefits are increasing making them more cost effective also. Thus another consideration for a heart failure specialist is to keep up with device technology advances. In practice, no one clinician will be capable in all the different areas mentioned and thus the ideal clinical management strategy is to be in the care of a multidisciplinary team. Such an approach with counseling support, specialist nursing support, device specialists, palliative care specialists, pharmacists, rehabilitation motivators and even finance advisors would be the ideal approach but such teams are rare and only likely to be affordable where critical mass of heart failure patients make that form of care equally affordable.

QUALITY IMPROVEMENT IN HEART FAILURE

Quality improvement initiatives in heart failure recommend community based approaches with specialist medical and palliative support services to reduce hospital admissions and optimise service provision [18]. An appointed health professional, possibly a specialist heart failure nurse, physician assistant or general practitioner could coordinate holistic care [74]. The British Heart Foundation recently provided funding for heart failure nurses specifically trained in palliative care and advanced communication skills [28] to fulfil this new role. A qualitative study with focus groups of medical professionals showed that many, if not most, doctors were enthusiastic about developing the role of the nurse in terminal heart failure. They described a 'superior ability of the nurse to liaise with other specialties and communicate with the patients and their relatives [31]. A community based approach such as this would also lead to improved integration with primary care.

Models of joint working have been developed, commonly with heart failure clinicians taking the lead role with palliative care colleagues in support [75]. One model of integrated care enabled half of patients to die at home with less than 10% requiring specific palliative care referral due to the 'ready availability of consultancy and systematic education activities and resources' [76]. Similar benefits have been seen in other UK regions such as Scarborough [77] and Bradford [78]. Going further, in Glasgow, the 'caring together' programme was launched in 2011 which involves the joint institutions of the Marie Curie Cancer Care, British Heart Foundation Scotland and NHS Greater Glasgow and Clyde working in partnership on a five-year programme, aiming to improve the quality and access to palliative care for any patients in the advanced stages of heart failure. The latest programme is developing an innovative approach to delivering palliative care for these patients in all care settings including hospital, hospice, care home and at home [79].

Hospice Use in Heart Failure

Hospice care for heart failure patients is on the rise slowly but surely, having been very limited in past decades. This care setting allows optimisation of heart failure care while also meeting the increasing palliative needs of patients and their partners as the heart failure progresses [19]. Evidence is readily available that the palliative needs of the patients are better addressed in a hospice rather than a hospital and there is some evidence to suggest that hospice care can even prolong the lives of patients in some cases [80]. Hospices are not only end stage placement but can also be for respite care for the partner or relatives who also have considerable psychosocial needs and mental fatigue. Varied levels of treatment are available in different hospices with some able to give treatment such as intravenous inotropes and continuous positive airways pressure (respiratory devices to improve oxygenation of lungs impaired by oedema) whilst others are limited to oral medications [81]. Hospices accept patients with devices but most still need to have in place, policies to manage devices at the end of life [82].

Patients should have the option of being referred to the appropriate hospice when their palliative care needs are significant and prognosis is poor. It is important however that the full capabilities of the hospice are disclosed so that patients and their families can make an informed decision about whether the hospice is right for them. The current USA guidelines recommend hospice admission as an option for end of life care in heart failure but the UK guidelines do not currently specify hospice care for these patients [5,18]. The numbers of patients that are referred to hospices for heart failure is currently poor with less than 5% of hospice patients being admitted for heart failure management [1, 83]. This further represents the lack of an integrated palliative approach in heart failure. It would be advantageous for clinicians to build relationships with local hospices to facilitate both transfer of patients to a hospice environment if required, and also to offer their on-going medical input and advice should the hospice staff need specialist input.

Economic Rationale for System Redesign

In the NHS heart failure survey in 2008 [84], there were approximately 9000 admissions across all hospital within one month, equating to 108,000 admissions and 16,200 death per year, with 2000 deaths occurring in the first two days of admission. An ideal situation of great benefit to patients and to hospitals, would be if these patients could be assessed in their own environments by a member of a community cardiac team. The patients could have immediate point of care tests in their homes allowing diagnosis with a BNP assay and calculation of a prediction score such as GWTG-HF score. With the help of this information and clinical examination, assessment could be made regarding patients' needs with appropriate onward triage to the best location for their further care. This may enable those who can be treated at home, while also identifying those needing hospital admission for acute care and those who would benefit from alternative location such as a hospice, for end stage symptom control. With an average inpatient length of stay of nine days prior to death in the large national audit [7], using this approach could potentially save nationally about 146,000 acute bed days per year, whilst also managing the most number of patients in the most suitable environment for their needs.

Role of Research in End of Life in Heart Failure

An additional consideration is that research is still limited in end of life heart failure, in part because of the difficulties of recruiting such ill patients into studies because such patients have numerous complication and confounding factors that prevent them being invited to or being eligible for research. Many studies for patients with end stage heart failure have failed to recruit to target citing low levels of interest and fear of therapies being experimental or harmful [85]. Thus advances in this field are slower than usual and less generalizable to the population of HF patients seen routinely. It is therefore critical to raise the profile of research in this field to ensure patients again don't have to deal with the complexities of being invited to research during difficult periods of decompensation of their HF but rather these options are discussed during initial or stable review consultations.

Summary

End of Life Care in Heart Failure patients has specific and special needs. The disease and its progression are unpredictable and various non-invasive and invasive therapies are available and need to be evaluated carefully with attention to the patient prognosis, benefit risk ratio, patient's quality of life, psychosocial wellbeing of patient and partner and the economy in which the care is occurring. Discussions need to be thorough and engaging without being depressing and overly complex. Patients need to be invited to consider advanced directives and express goals and psychosocial needs. Physicians need to be trained to have a holistic approach as well as considering the wide range of treatments available in HF for both disease management and symptom control.

Palliative and community care teams need to be engaged early on and risk scores to understand patient prognosis from the outset of meeting the patient should be considered. When offering complex device therapies, early discussion of treatment withdrawal or deactivation of certain components needs to happen to prepare for more difficult times. Specialist nurses and physician assistants may be best to handle monitoring of care and to broach the psychosocial needs. Hospice and homes need to be considered as appropriate locations for care as appropriate and a multidisciplinary approach needs to be formulated for more complex HF patients. In summary, HF which is both a long term chronic condition and a difficult to manage disease needs to be approached with respect and consideration of the many complexities that may arise. It also requires a very positive or detached approach given the emotional impact the diagnosis of HF can have on patients, carers and even the clinicians managing such patients.

REFERENCES

[1] Levenson, JW; McCarthy, EP; Lynn, J. et al. the last six months of life for patients with congestive cardiac failure. *J Am Geriatr Soc*, 2000, 48 (5 suppl), S101-S109.

[2] Lehman, R; Doust, J; Glasziou, P. Cardiac impairment or heart failure? *BMJ*, 2005, 331(7514), 415-416.

[3] www.heartstats.org (The Bristish Heart Foundation statistics website).

[4] Lloyd-Jones, D; Adams, RJ; Brown, TM; et al. Heart Disease and Stroke Statistics 2010 Update. A Report From the American Heart Association. *Circulation*, 2010, 121, e46-e215.

[5] Heart Failure Society of America. Evaluation and management of patients with acute decompensated heart failure. *J Card Fail*, 2006, 12, e86-e103.

[6] Rose, EA; Moskowitz, AJ; Packer, M; et al. The REMATCH trial, rationale, design, and end points. Randomized Evaluation of Mechanical Assistance for the Treatment of Congestive Heart Failure. *Ann Thorac Surg*, 1999, 67, 723-730.

[7] NHS Modernisation Agency. Coronary heart disease collaborative, palliaitive and supportive care in heart failure. http://www.improvement.nhs.uk/heart/Portals/0/documents/supportive and palliativecare.pdf.

[8] Rector, TS. A conceptual model of quality of life in relation to heart failure. *J Card Fail*, 2005, 11, 173-6.

[9] Rector, TS; Tschumperlin, LK; Kubo, SH; et al. Use of the living with heart failure questionnaire to ascertain patients' perspectives on improvement in quality of life versus risk of drug induced death. *J Card Fail*, 1995, 1, 201-6.

[10] Barnes, S; Gott, M; Payne, S; Parker, C; Seamark, D; Gariballa, S; Small, N. Prevelance of symptoms in a community based sample of heart failure patients. *J Pain Symptom Manage*, 2006, 32, 208-21.

[11] Bekelman, D; Havranek, E; Becker, D; Kutner, J; Peterson, P; Wittstein, I; Gottlieb, S; Yamashita, T; Fairclough, D; Dy, S. Symptoms, depression, and quality of life in patients with heart failure. *J Card Fail*, 2007, 13, 643-648.

[12] Kirkpatrick, JN; Guger, CJ; Arnsdorf, MF; Fedson, SE. Advance directives in the cardiac care unit. *Am Heart J*, 2007, 154(3), 477-481

[13] NHS Information Centre. National Heart Failure Audit 2010. Leeds, National Clinical Audit Support Programme, 2010.

[14] Anderson, H; Ward, C; Gomm, SA; Connolly, M; Coppinger, T; Corgie, D; Williams, JL; Makin, WP. The concerns of patients under palliative care and a heart failure clinic are not being met. *Pall Med*, 2001, 15, 279-286.

[15] Murray, S; Boyd, K; Kendall, M; Worth, A; Benton, TF; Clausen, H. Dying of lung cancer or cardiac failure, prospective qualitative interview study of patients and their carers in the community. *BMJ*, 2002, 325, 929.

[16] NHS Modernisation Agency. Supportive and palliative care for advanced heart failure. Leicester, NHS Modernisation Agency 2004.

[17] Department of Health. *National service framework for coronary heart disease*. London, DOH 2000.

[18] National Institute for Health and Clinical Excellence. Management of chronic heart failure in adults in primary and secondary care. London, *National Institute for Health and Clinical Excellence*, 2010.

[19] Department of Health, End of life care strategy for adults. London, DOH 2008.
[20] Department of Health. *End of life care strategy*, 2st annual report. www.dh.gov.uk/en/Publicationsandstatistics/Publications/PublicationsPolicyAndGuidance/DH_118810.
[21] http://www.gmccsn.nhs.uk/files/8113/6983/8277/ICD_Deactivation_PolicyFinal_V1.0.pdf.
[22] http://www.slcsn.nhs.uk/files/cardiac/sl-guidelines-icd-deactivation-012013.pdf.
[23] Harding, R; Selman, L; Beynon, T; et al. Meeting the communication and information needs of chronic heart failure patients. *J Pain Symptom M*, 2008, 36, 149-156.
[24] Kirkpatrick, JN; Guger, CJ; Arnsdorf, MF; Fedson, SE. Advance directives in the cardiac care unit. *Am Heart J*, 2007, 154, 477-481.
[25] Habal, MV; Micevski, V; Greenwood, S; et al. How aware of advance care directives are heart failure patients, and are they using them? *Can J Cardiol*, 2011, 27, 376-381.
[26] Lewis, EF; Johnson, PA; Johnson, W; Collins, C; Griffin, L; Stevenson, LW. Preferences for quality of life or survival expressed by patients with heart failure. *Journal of heart and lung transplantation*, 2001, 20, 9, 101-1024.
[27] Krumholz, HM; Phillips, RS; Hamel, MB; et al. Resuscitation preferences among patients with severe congestive heart failure, results from the SUPPORT project. *Circulation*, 1998, 98, 7, 648-655.
[28] Jaarsma, T; Beattie, J; Ryder, M; Rutten, F; McDonagh, T; Mohacsi, P; et al. Palliative care in heart failure, a position statement from the palliative care workshop of the Heart Failure Association of the European Society of Cardiology. *Eur J Heart Failure*, 2009, 11, 433-443.
[29] Rogers, A; Addlington-Hall, J; McCoy, A; Edmonds, P; Abery, A; Coats, A; Gibbs, J. A qualitative study on chronic heart failure patients' understanding of their symptoms and drug therapy. *Eur J Heart Failure*, 2002, 4, 283-287.
[30] Koelling, TM; Johnson, ML; Cody, RJ; Aaronson, KD. Discharge education improves clinical outcomes in patients with chronic heart failure. *Circulation*, 2005, 111, 179-185.
[31] Hanratty, B; Hibbert, D; Mair, F; May, C; Ward, C; Capewell, S; Litva, A; Corcoran, G. Doctors' perceptions of palliative care for heart failure, focus group study. *BMJ*, 2002, 325, 581-5.

[32] Nordgren, L; Olsson, H. Palliative care in a coronary care unit, a qualitiative study of physicians' and nurses' perceptions. *J Clin Nurs*, 2004, 13, 185-193.
[33] Selman, L; Harding, R; Beynon, T; et al. Improving end of life care for patients with chronic heart failure, 'let's hope it'll get better when I know in my heart it won't'. *Heart*, 2007, 93(8), 963-967.
[34] World Health Organisation website http://www.who.int/cancer/palliative/en/
[35] Maguire, P; Pitceathley, C. Key communication skills and how to acquire them. *Br Med J*, 2002, 325, 697-700.
[36] Heffner, J; Barbieri, C. End of life preferences for patients enrolled in heart failure rehabilitation programmes. *Chest*, 2000, 117(5), 1474-1481.
[37] Wright, AA; Zhang, B; Ray, A; et al. Associations between end of life discussions, patient mental health, medical care near death and caregiver bereavement adjustment. *JAMA*, 2008, 300, 1665-1673.
[38] Levy, WC; Mozaffarian, D; Linker, DT; et al. The Seattle Heart Failure Model. Prediction of survival in heart failure. *Circulation*, 2006, 113, 1424-1433.
[39] Peterson, PN; Rumsfeld, JS; Liang, L; et al. A validation risk score for in-hospital mortality in patients with heart failure from the American Heart Association Get With the Guidelines Programme. *Cir cCardiovasc Qual Outcomes*, 2010, 3, 00-00.
[40] Fonarow, GC; Adams, KF Jr; Abraham, WT; Yancy, CW; Boscardin, WJ for the ADHERE Scientific Advisory CommoitteeSGaI. Risk stratification for in-hospital mortality in acutely decompensated heart failure, classification and regression tree analysis. *JAMA*, 2005, 293, 572-580.
[41] Ky, B; French, B; Levy, WC; et al. Multiple biomarkers for risk prediction in chronic heart failure. *Circ Heart Fail*, 2012, 5, 183-90.
[42] Bjurman, C; Jensen, J; Petzold, M; et al. Assessment of a multimarker strategy for prediction of mortality in older heart failure patients, a cohort study. BMJ open 2013, 3, e002254 Paper 5 ref 3 Stevenson LW, The Evolving Role of Mechanical Circulatory Support in Advanced Heart Failure. ISHLT Monograph Series 2006. 1 Chapter 11, 181-204.
[43] Bekelman, DB; Rumsfeld, JS; Havranek, EP; et al. Symptom burden, depression and spiritual well being, a comparison of heart failure and advanced cancer patients. *J Gen Intern Med*, 2009, 24, 592-598.

[44] Thomas, K. The Gold Standards Framework, A Programme for community palliative care. London, Department of Health 2005. Available at http, //www.goldstandardsframework.nhs.uk.

[45] National Heart Failure Audit – Fifth Annual report published 27th Nov 2012. www.ucl.ac.uk/nicor/audits/heartfailure/additionalfiles/pdfs/ annualreports/annual12.pdf.

[46] Steel, A; Bakhai, A. Proposal for routine use of mortality risk prediction tools to promote early end of life planning in heart failure patients and facilitate integrated care. *Int J Cardiol.*, 2013 Jul 15, 167(1), 280-2. doi, 10.1016/j.ijcard.2012.09.211. Epub 2012 Nov 27.

[47] Stevenson, LW. The Evolving role of Mechanical Circulatory support in Advanced Heart Failure. *ISHLT Monograph series*, 2006, 1 chapter 11, 181-204.

[48] Rogers, JG; Butler, J; Lansman, SL; et al. Chronic mechanical circulatory support for ionotrope dependent heart failure patients who are not transplant candidates, results of the INTrEPID trial. *J Am Coll Cardiol*, 2007, 50, 741-747.

[49] Fields, AV; Kirkpatrick, JN. Ethics of the Heart, Ethical and Policy Challenges in the Treatment of Advanced Heart Failure. *Perspectives in Biology and Medicine*, 2012, 55(1), 71-80.

[50] Kirkpatrick, JN; Fedson, SE; Verdino, R. Ethical dilemmas in device treatment for advanced heart failure. *Curr Opin Support Palliat Care*, 2007, 1, 267-273.

[51] Jarman, JW; Lascelles, K; Wong, T; Markides, V; Clague, JR; Till, J. Clinical experience of entirely subcutaneous implantable cardioverter-defibrillators in children and adults, cause for caution. *Eur Heart J.*, 2012 Jun, 33(11), 1351-9.

[52] Olde Nordkamp, LR; Dabiri Abkenari, L; Boersma, LV; Maass, AH; de Groot, JR; van Oostrom, AJ; Theuns, DA; Jordaens, LJ; Wilde, AA; Knops, RE. The entirely subcutaneous implantable cardioverter-defibrillator, initial clinical experience in a large Dutch cohort. *J Am Coll Cardiol.*, 2012 Nov 6, 60(19), 1933-9.

[53] Cleland, JG; Daubert, JC; Erdmann, E; et al. The effect of cardiac resynchronization on morbidity and mortality in heart failure. *N Engl J Med*, 2005, 352, 1539-1549.

[54] Yu, CM; Wing-Hong Fung, J; Zhang, Q; Sanderson, JE. Understanding nonresponders of cardiac resynchronization therapy--current and future perspectives. *J Cardiovasc Electrophysiol.*, 2005 Oct, 16(10), 1117-24.

[55] Park, SJ; Milano, CA; Tatooles, AJ; et al. Outcomes in advanced heart failure patients with left ventricular assist devices for destination therapy. *Circ Heart Fail*, 2012, 5, 241-248.
[56] Smith, T; Jordaens, L; Theuns, DA; et al. The cost-effectiveness of primary prophylactic implantable defibrillator therapy in patients with ischemic or non-ischemic heart disease, an European analysis. *Eur Heart J*, 2013 Jan, 34(3), 211-9.
[57] Rogers, JG; Bostic, RR; Tong, KB; et al. Cost-effectiveness analysis of continuous-flow left ventricular assist devices as destination therapy. *Circ Heart Fail*, 2012, 5, 10-16.
[58] Grimes, DS. Rationing health care. *Lancet*, 1987. 1(8533), 615-616.
[59] Hope, T; Reynolds, J; Griffiths, S. Rationing decisions, integrating cost effectiveness with other values. Medicine and Social Justice, *Essays on the Distribution of Health Care*. R Rhodes, M Battin and A Silvers, EDS 144-155, Oxford Universit Press, New York 2002.
[60] La Puma, J; Lawlor, EF. Quality-Adjusted Life-Years Ethical Implications for Physicians and Policymakers. *JAMA*., 1990, 263(21), 2917-2921.
[61] Harris, J. QALYfying the value of life. *Journal of Medical Ethics*, 1987. 13(3), 117-123.
[62] Goldstein, NE; Lampert, R; Bradley, E; et al. Management of implantable cardioverter defibrillators in end-of-life care. *Ann Intern Med*, 2004, 141, 835-838.
[63] Fromme, EK; Stewart, TL; Jeppesen, M; Tolle, SW. Adverse experiences with implantable defibrillators in Oregon hospices. *Am J Hosp Palliat Care*., 2011 Aug, 28(5), 304-9.
[64] Raphael, CE; Koa-Wing, M; Stain, N; et al. Implantable cardioverter-defibrillator recipient attitudes towards device deactivation, how much do patients want to know? *Pacing Clin Electrophysiol*, 2011, 34, 1628-1633.
[65] Long, JW; Kfoury, AG; Slaughter, MS; et al. Long term destination therapy with the Heart-Mate XVE left ventricular assist device, improved outcomes since the REMATCH study. *Congest Heart Fail*., 2005, 11, 133-138.
[66] Sulmasy, DP. Within you/without you, biotechnology, ontology, and ethics. *J Gen Intern Med*., 2008, 23 Suppl 1, 69-72.
[67] Carlsson, J; Paul, NW; Dann, M; Neuzner, J; Pfeiffer, D. The deactivation of implantable cardioverter-defibrillators, medical, ethical,

practical, and legal considerations. *Dtsch Arztebl Int.*, 2012 Aug, 109(33-34), 535-41.

[68] England, R; England, T; Coggon, J. The ethical and legal implications of deactivating an implantable cardioverter-defibrillator in a patient with terminal cancer. *J Med Ethics*, 2007, 33, 538-540.

[69] Kay, GN; Bittner, GT. Should implantable cardioverter-defibrillators and permanent pacemakers in patients with terminal illness be deactivated? Deactivating implantable cardioverter-defibrillators and permanent pacemakers in patients with terminal illness. An ethical distinction. *Circ Arrhythmia Electrophysiol.*, 2009, 2, 336-339.

[70] Mueller, PS; Swetz, KM; Freeman, MR; et al. Ethical analysis of withdrawing ventricular assist device support. *Mayo Clin Proc*, 2010, 85, 791-797.

[71] Singer, PA; Robertson, G; Roy, DJ. Bioethics for clinicians, Advance care planning. *CAMJ*, 1996, 155, 1689-92.

[72] Mezu, U; Adelstein, E; Jain, S; Saba, S. Effectiveness of implantable defibrillators in octogenerians and nonagenarians for primary prevention of sudden cardiac death. *Am J Cardiol*, 2011, 108, 718-722.

[73] Petrucci, RJ; Benish, LA; Carrow, BL; et al. Ethical considerations for ventricular assist device support, a 10-point model. *ASAIO J*, 2011, 57, 268-273.

[74] Boyd, K; Worth, A; Kendall, M; Pratt, R; Hockley, J; Denvir, M; Murray, S. Making sure services deliver for people with advanced heart failure, a longitudinal qualitative study of patients, family carers, and health professionals. *Pall Med*, 2009, 23(8), 767-776.

[75] Daley, A; Matthews, C; Williams, A. Heart Failure and palliative care services working in partnership, report of a new model of care. *Pall Med*, 2006, 20(6), 593-601.

[76] Davidson, P; Paull, G; Introna, K; Cockburn, J; Davis, J; Rees, D; et al. Integrated. Collaborative Pallaitive Care in Heart Failure. *J Cardiovasc Nursing*, 2004, 19(1), 68-75.

[77] Johnson, M; Houghton, T. Palliative care for patients with heart failure, description of a service. *Pall Med*, 2006, 20, 211-214.

[78] Daley, A; Matthews, C; Williams, A. Heart Failure and palliative care services working in partnership, report of a new model of care. *Pall Med*, 2006, 20, 593-601.

[79] http://www.mariecurie.org.uk/en-GB/Commissioners-and-referrers/Partnerships-and-innovations/Caring-together/

[80] Goodlin, SJ; Kutner, JS; Connor, SR; et al. Hospice care for heart failure patients. *J Pain Symptom Manage*, 2005, 29, 525-528.

[81] Pantilat, SZ; Steimle, AE. Palliative care for patients with heart failure. *JAMA*, 2004, 291, 2476-2482.

[82] Goodlin, SJ; Kutner, JS; Connor, SR; et al. Hospice care for heart failure patients. *J Pain Symptom Manag*, 29, 525-28.

[83] Connor, SR; Pyenson, B; Fitch, K; et al. Comparing hospice and non-hospice patient survival among patients who die within a three year window. *J Pain Symptom Manage*, 2007, 33, 238-246.

[84] Russo, MJ; Gelijins, AC; Stevenson, LW; et al., The cost of medical management in advanced heart failure during the final two years of life. *J Card Fail*, 2008, 14, 651-658.

[85] Zambroski, CH; Buck, H; Garrison, CM; McMillan, SC. Lessons From the Field, Challenges in Accruing Hospice Heart Failure Patients to Intervention Research. *J Cardiovasc Nurs*., 2013 Feb 14.

In: End-of-Life Care
Editors: Maria Rossi and Luiz Ortiz
ISBN: 978-1-62808-555-6

Chapter 2

END-OF-LIFE EXPERIENCES: A SPIRITUAL PERSPECTIVE

Peter Fenwick
Maudsley Hospital London.
Institute of Psychiatry, King's College, London, UK

ABSTRACT

Spiritual awareness is an important part of care for the dying. Our research with a palliative care team, and with the carers in hospices and a nursing home, has confirmed that end-of-life experiences, which occur in the last few days of life have spiritual implications for the dying and their families, and are not uncommon. These experiences include visions by the dying, usually of dead relatives, deathbed 'coincidences', in which someone emotionally close to a dying person reports being 'visited' by them at the time of their death, and the feeling of going into and out of another reality. Carers of the dying also report that at the moment of death they may see something leaving the body or light surrounding it. Carers also report the desire which the dying often show for reconciliation with their life and, importantly other family members. Nearly all the reports (85%) suggested that these experiences are profoundly comforting both to the dying themselves, and to any family members who witness the phenomena.

The study has clear implications for theories about the continuation of consciousness after death. New studies on after-death experiences during cardiac arrest, in which patients report seeing the resuscitation process, suggest that our current model of brain function may need to be expanded. One interpretation of the data is that it may point to a continuation of consciousness.

INTRODUCTION

Most of us are afraid of death. As Freud observed, when we talk about it, we always talk about other people's death, never our own. The need to care for the dying, to minimise pain and suffering and provide a safe, loving environment in which the dying can be cared for, must be our primary concern. But we need to recognise, too, that dying is a very spiritual time, and the spiritual needs and experiences of the dying are perhaps less generally recognised, and certainly less well catered for. Finally, and for this article most importantly, dying is a time when consciousness is lost, the psychic life of the individual ends, and they are taken out of the web of relationships that they have formed during their life. It is this aspect of death which has essentially been overlooked in our culture, and it is to this, and to the spiritual nature of dying, that this chapter will direct most attention .

That death and dying are seldom discussed is also a matter of concern for some medical practitioners. Seravalli states that doctors and nurses are often adversely affected by death, either because they themselves fear death and identify with the dying person, or because they feel professionally impotent in the face of it. He maintains, however, that if we can understand better the particular world of the dying, these feelings might become bearable [1]. This supposition echoes the findings of Elizabeth Kubler Ross who, during her extensive research into the dying process, found in medical staff not only denial and rationalisation of these experiences, but also hostility and even aggressive behaviour. She concluded, "What all of us have to learn is to accept death as part of life. When we have learned this, then maybe we can help our patients learn it too" [2]. Heyse-Morse also stressed the need to consider the spiritual pain of dying, and the importance of the right kind of support given by the carer. He believed "Effective help implies that the carer is fully present to the sufferer, person to person, deep calling to deep".[3]. In a random stratified survey in the USA patients, family, physicians and other care providers were asked to rate factors that they considered important at the end-of-life. Pain and symptom management, preparation for death and achieving a sense of completion were all high on the list. A number of items received strong importance ratings from patients. Amongst these were being mentally aware and coming to peace with God. Clearly, an understanding of the death process, remaining mentally in touch and help with spiritual conflicts were all important [4].

MENTAL STATES OF THE DYING

The mental states of the dying have received only little attention. For the dying, they map a path that they may go through in the dying process. For the family they can be and frequently are a source of enormous comfort, and for our culture, they give us some understanding of the way that consciousness is lost and possibly even allow us a glimpse into the future, and what may lie there.

Anecdotal accounts of, and phenomena associated with, approaching death have been noted for many centuries and in many cultures. These anecdotal accounts suggest that death may be heralded by premonitions that you or someone you love is going to die, and by phenomena such as visions, or apparitions, that comfort the dying person and prepare them spiritually for death, or for the 'crossing over' to a new reality.

STUDIES OF END-OF-LIFE EXPERIENCES

In 2004 Sue Brayne, a palliative care worker, and I set out to find whether end-of-life experiences did indeed occur, and if so, how common were they and what was their phenomenology. We started the process by questioning a palliative care team and this showed us the divisions between medical and nursing staff, and care workers [5]. The medical staff were very hesitant to admit to the existence of these experiences. The nurses and care-workers had come across many examples, and these were discussed more freely by the care-workers than the nursing staff. On the basis of this data we formulated a questionnaire which we gave to hospice and nursing home care-workers both in the UK and Holland. We learned that many of the nurses and care-workers were unaware of the full range of end-of-life experiences, so we decided to ask them what experiences they had come across in the previous five years (5-year retrospective) and then to ask them to keep a record and note the experiences that they came across in the next year (one-year prospective) [6]. We also collected data from the general public about end-of-life experiences, and have over 1000 accounts of these experiences.

DEATH BED VISIONS

These are perhaps the most commonly reported end-of-life experiences (ELEs). The visions are usually seen in clear, or only moderately impaired, consciousness [7-9] are usually of dead relatives, frequently someone the dying person had a close emotional contact with and they usually respond to their visitors with interest and joy. They seem to provide comfort and reassurance at this crucial time in the dying process. The 'visitor' may first appear outside the dying person's window or the room but gradually move closer and often just before death sit on their bed.

Although many visions are seen within about 12 hours of death, they often occur days or even weeks before. In our series of 45 accounts, 8% said the experience occurred more than a week before death, 26% within seven days of death, 8% within 24 hours, but the majority- 54% - occurred in the 12 hours before death. Of those people who experienced the DBV , 62% were dying, 9% were severely ill but not expected to die, and 14%, although ill, were not severely ill and death was quite unexpected. The final 14% had been in coma but aroused and had the experience during this brief period of lucidity

Occasionally the experience occurs even to someone who seems perfectly well. In one such account a daughter describes how one day her mother popped in to visit her grandmother who told her:

> "'I can't understand it! I just saw my mother standing in the doorway, as clearly as I can see you.' She goes on: "....At that time my grandmother was no more ill than she had been for the last two or three years and perfectly lucid...The next day, my grandmother suffered a massive stroke from which she never regained consciousness. After lying in a coma for four days, she died".

The visions are not dependent on religious belief or expectation, though their content may be culturally influenced. In our sample 70% saw dead relatives or friends, most commonly siblings, parents or spouses. Only 3% described angels and no other religious figures were seen. Nearly all saw a single apparition. 11% saw two or more, while 16% saw three or more.

One practicing Catholic correspondent, whose father saw angels, commented:

> "....this sort of phenomenon has nothing to do with our Faith. We were all as surprised as anyone of any faith or no faith would be"

The visions are seen in real space. The dying person's eyes seem to look fixedly at a particular point, or to follow someone who is apparently moving around the room. Often they interact with them, and expect others to do so too. A nurse described how, with a fellow nurse, she was attending a dying patient.

> "The patient asked us to stand one on each side of him because he wanted to thank us for looking after him. He then looked over my shoulder towards the window and said 'hang on I will be with you in a minute, I just want to thank these nurses for looking after me'. The patient repeated himself a couple of times then died!"

Our own findings confirmed those of Osis and Haraldsson [7] that there is often a change in mood just before death which is not attributable to medication or medical factors.

> "She suddenly sat up in bed her arms out towards someone with a great look of happiness and then after a pause sank back on the pillow and died not long after."

And again another account.

> "Suddenly my Gran sat up in bed and smiled. She said "I'm going now and here's Dad and George come to meet me". She then died still with this big smile on her face. My mother never forgot it."

Carers say that quite often a patient's language will change after they have had one of these visions. They start to use 'journeying' language saying that they won't be here tomorrow, – they are going to be taken or collected, are going away, will be on a journey. 33% said the experience was comforting and reassuring to the patient, and 51% described the dying as being very happy to see their visitor. The apparition helped the dying to let go of life in 8% of cases. However, 9% were said to be confused by the experience, though only one person in the whole sample found the apparition frightening or distressing. Most importantly, family members who witnessed these experiences also found them comforting.

Transiting to a New Reality

About 48% of the carers in our study told us that in the period just before death patients seem to move in and out of a new reality, which seems just as real, often more real, than the room in which they are , and is interpenetrated by light, love and compassion. Within this area they experience a widening of their spiritual vision and see spiritual beings who they don't know but whose purity is strongly evident.. Sometimes the patient's consciousness will move into this new reality and linger there, at others it is a short, transient look. This reality is very similar to that described in the near death experience, except that the dead relatives they meet say they are there to meet them and help them through the dying process. Although relatives are most often met, strangers and spiritual beings are also sometimes seen, but all are experienced as a comforting presence, there to help with the dying process and holding out the promise of the possibility of a continuation of consciousness.

The patient then returns to their room and is sometimes surprised that they have come back. These visits are very reassuring to the patient who is then able to reassure those caring for them that they will be all right when they die and there is no need to worry about them..

The mother of a 32 yr old woman dying of breast cancer described to me what happened in the last two to three days of her daughter's life..

> "She was conscious of a dark roof over her head and a bright light. She moved into a waiting place where beings, her grandfather amongst them, were there to help her and told her everything would be ok. She moved into and out of this area, and was adamant that it was not a dream."

Something Leaving the Body

The perception of something leaving the body around the time of death is a little discussed phenomenon, and we did not ask about its frequency in our survey. However, we have had many anecdotal reports from the general public. The accounts are very varied, but central to this experience is a form or shape which may leave the body, usually from the mouth, chest or through the head though we have also had accounts of something leaving through the feet. Sometimes it will hover above the body before rising to disappear through the ceiling and it is often associated with love, light, compassion. Not everyone who is in the room sees the vision, its appearance is transient and its perception is sensitive to interruption - people coming into the room or talking often make it disappear. It is enormously comforting to any of the bereaved who have the experience and may remain a comfort over many years.

> "Suddenly there was the most brilliant light shining from my husband's chest and as this light lifted upwards there was the most beautiful music and singing voices, my own chest seemed filled with infinite joy and my heart felt as if it was lifting to join this light and music. Suddenly there was a hand on my shoulder and a nurse said "I'm sorry love. He has just gone." I lost sight of the light and music, I felt so bereft at being left behind."

These phenomena can occur anywhere, not only in a hospice. We have an account of a shape seen leaving the body of a man who had just died of a heart attack on a golf course. The GP who rushed to help gave an account of the shape he saw leaving the man's body after his death. We have another account from a forester who was working with a colleague cutting down trees. A piece of equipment fell and crushed his colleague and killed him. The forester then describes the slow rising of a shape out of the body and disappearing

These shapes are sometimes described as like a wavering heat haze, sometimes as smoke-like, sometimes with a more definite form and appearing more solid, when they are usually accompanied by light. They have been described as 'soul mist' although the term is unsatisfactory as many are not mist-like. Not everyone present may see the shape, but those who do have little doubt that they have seen the soul leaving the body and find it comforting as they take it as an indication of the movement of consciousness to elsewhere..

DEATHBED COINCIDENCES (DBC)

There are many reports by someone emotionally close to a dying person of an awareness of that person's death, even though they may be at a distance from them and not even know they are ill. Over 50% of the carers in our study have had been told of these experiences by relatives so they are not uncommon.[10]. In a detailed analysis of 45 DBC 80% were experienced by a first-degree relative of the dying, granddaughters and grandmothers being the largest group at 17%. In 93% the experience was verified within three days of the death as occurring at the time of death. Death was unexpected in 44% of the cases. 27% were said to be ill and 17% to be dying. In 11% of cases death was swift, as the result of a violent accident.

These experiences are short lasting and the form they take will depend on the mental state of the person 'visited'. If they are awake (35% of our sample) they may have an overwhelming and inexplicable wave of emotion on which they feel compelled to act, or conviction that something has happened to the person, or simply an awareness of their presence, perhaps with the feeling that they have come to say goodbye. If they are asleep the visit will be a much more explicit, usually in the form of a narrative dream (26%), or immediately on waking from sleep and is associated with feelings of love, light and compassion: they will see the person who indicates that they have come to say goodbye, and often to tell them they must not worry. 38% of our sample were asleep, but made no mention of a dream. When apparitions do appear they do so whole, and as if they were in the prime of life. 32% received a warning that the sender was dying or had died. However, in 49% they had come to say farewell and reassure the recipient that they were all right.

> "When I retired to bed .... I tossed this way and that until suddenly in the early hours my father stood by my bed. He had been ill for a long time, but there he was standing in his prime of life. He didn't speak. My restlessness ceased and I fell asleep. In the morning I knew... my father had died late the evening before and had been permitted to visit me on his way into the next life." (Personal communication)

Radiant Light

Between 30% and 50% of carers report the presence of radiant light either surrounding the body or in the room at the time of death. This light is frequently described as full of love and compassion.

> "Suddenly there was the most brilliant light shinig from my husband's chest and as this light lifted upwards there was the most beautiful music and singing voices, my own chest seemed filled with infinite joy and my heart felt as if it was lifting to join this light and

music. Suddenly there was a hand on my shoulder and a nurse said 'I'm sorry love. He has just gone.' I felt so bereft at being left behind." [9]

TERMINAL LUCIDITY

Since the 18th Century it has been noted that immediately before death patients may suddenly alert from coma, often say goodbye to their relatives before sinking back into the bed and dying. In Victorian times this was called 'lightening up before death' and was explained as allowing the dying to have a brief moment with their relatives before death supervened. Current assessment suggests that its frequency is about 6% and that the degree of lightening depends on the patient but it is always sufficient for the person to enter clear consciousness and recognise his family. In the last few years there have been accounts of patients who were mentally ill, demented or suffering from brain damage who have become lucid, perhaps for the first time for years, just before their death. No scientific explanation for this phenomenon has yet been found but it raises intriguing questions. [11]

RESPONSE OF CARERS TO END-OF-LIFE EXPERIENCES

Although many carers find ELEs hard to explain or to define clinically, most agree that they are an intensely personal - and often a spiritual – experience, helping the patient to become reconciled with events in their life, and therefore to come to terms with their death. 78% of the carers in our sample were convinced of the validity of the experience; 11% were not sure of its true meaning and only one person was sceptical [10]. But even though our studies have found that most carers are aware of end-of-life phenomena, they did not always find it easy to know how to respond to patients who experienced them. And it also became clear that the patients themselves were often reluctant to talk about them, either through embarrassment, fear that they wouldn't be believed, or thought mad, or simply through inadequacy of language to describe the experiences. Patients are not asked routinely about their experiences by medical and nursing staff, medical training is not conducive to encouraging patients to talk, and some patients may simply not want to talk about their ELEs.

We have also found that many palliative care workers are acutely aware of, and challenged by, being viewed as spiritual mentors who can provide answers to searching questions, or confirm the patient's own beliefs. Current training for palliative workers does not specifically prepare them to deal with the pastoral needs of the dying.

Openness and honesty, a willingness to listen, and an ability to understand a patient's language or signals will all encourage patients to speak of ELE experiences. Often patients simply need to be reassured that their experiences are quite normal and happen to quite a few people, most of whom find it comforting. They also need to 'test the waters'. "*Patients.... might tell you half of something. They want to know whether you are okay with that. Then they might tell you a bit more*"

EXPLANATORY MODELS

Now that the evidence points to a wide range of phenomena occurring in the days before and at the time of death, we need to widen the usual medical model of death to a broader model which is able to encompasses these phenomena. Clearly deathbed coincidences, if confirmed by other workers, would suggest that the dying mind is somehow extended, and this suggestion maps on to some of the scientific findings concerning non-local mind. Although the idea of non-local mind is alien to those of us who were brought up with the classical materialistic reductionist framework, when looking for an explanation for ELEs we need to look at the evidence which may point to mind being extended. Although a detailed discussion of this is beyond the scope of this article, there are a number of studies which suggest that mind beyond the brain is a possibility which now needs to be taken seriously. The following are some examples - prayer [12] telepathy [13], and distant healing [14].

The closest science has come to understanding the actual subjective process of dying is through studying the near death experience. This is a complex and controversial area, but it becomes clearer if the correct model for the NDE is chosen. Dr Sam Parnia and I chose the cardiac arrest model as patients in the UK are resuscitated in accordance with a fixed protocol. So we can be certain that when the heart stops the physiological processes occurring in the brain are the same in every case. These experiences were called NDEs but because of the timing and their relation to cardiac arrest they are best called after death experience, ADEs. There are now five major studies of ADEs which have occurred in cardiac arrest [15-19]. There is a strong consensus that drugs or anoxia are not the cause of these experiences. Indeed, it has been difficult to find a reductionist explanation that sits happily with the neuroscience evidence that at the time the experience was occurring the patient's brain was dead, and the functioning was disturbed to such an extent so as to be unable to support consciousness.

Within 11 to 17 seconds of a cardiac arrest the EEG flatlines, the patient's pupils dilate, the cough reflex goes, they stop breathing. These are all signs of death. It is true that the patient can be resuscitated, but nevertheless the death process has begun. Physiologically, the lack of oxygen to the brain leads to an inability of the neurones to replenish their energy stores. As soon as the ATP (adenosine triphosphate) stores are exhausted the cell enters a phase during which it is unable to maintain the integrity of the cell membrane which is crucial for it to function. Calcium now enters the cell together with ions of sodium and potassium and this initiates an excito-toxic process which will eventually lead to the cell's destruction. If this process goes on for any length of time beyond four to five minutes the damage which has occurred may be so great that normal function cannot easily be re-established and significant brain damage will occur if the heart restarts. Thus it is necessary to take very seriously accounts that some people have given of conscious experience during the period when the brain is not functioning. Accounts of the cardiac arrest experiences suggest that in about a third of the ten percent of cases in which the ADE occurs after cardiac arrest, the patient reports that he leaves his body and watches the resuscitation process from a vantage point on the ceiling. These experiences are called Veridical ADEs and over one hundred have been recorded and verified [20]. If the resuscitation process is prolonged the patient may go down a tunnel toward the light, meet a Being of Light and then into a Paradise –like area where they will meet their dead relatives, may have a life review and - provided the heart restarts – will then return to their bodies. These ADEs are very similar to the NDE occurring in other situations, but it is important to keep the two sets of experiences separate, as in the ADE we know precisely the state of the brain's physiology and so can be much more certain that these experiences are truly occurring when brain function is no longer possible because of lack of oxygen and the cellular degradation processes which have already commenced.

First, it cannot be argued that these experiences occur either before the cardiac arrest and unconsciousness, or after heart function has been resumed and the patient is able to distinguish the timing of the experience. In practice the initial loss of consciousness is very rapid. The patient is fully aware up to the moment when consciousness is lost and thus the experiences cannot occur at this time. Because of the disruption to cellular function which resulted from the cardiac arrest, recovery is always confusional. But the ADE is not confusional but lucid, with a strong emotional content. Thus it is unlikely to have occurred during the confusional state after the heart has re-started. This leaves the period of unconsciousness as the most likely time for the experience to have occurred, the time when the patients also say it did.

Next, as already mentioned, approximately a third of the patients who have an ADE during cardiac arrest report leaving their bodies and watching the resuscitation process. It is argued that their accounts are similar to what actually happened during the arrest, because television has led us to have an approximate idea of the process. This theory was tested by Sartori, who is an intensive care nurse who carried out a study for her post-doctoral thesis of ADEs during cardiac arrest. She divided her sample of patients into those who had a cardiac arrest and no OBE and those who did report leaving their body. She asked both groups to describe what happened during the resuscitation. The group who had seen it gave a much more accurate description than the group who had not: moreover the descriptions given by those who had not had the OBE indicated little understanding of cardiac arrest treatment. This suggests that the patient had truly been able to obtain information about the arrest and treatment process when they were unconsciousness [19].

Finally, it is argued that there are small areas of the brain which are still functioning during the arrest and thus ordinary sensations such as hearing and vision are still present, and it is memory of these which has been reconstructed into the out of body experience. However, this view fails to understand the physiological processes necessary in the brain for a conscious experience to arise. As I have mentioned, within 11-17 seconds cortical activity is no longer measurable as the EEG has flatlined and severe brain stem dysfunction has occurred. Within the brain stem is located the reticular activating system which needs to be fully functional if the cortex of the brain is to maintain conscious experience. The reticular activating system drives the non-specific nuclei of the thalamus and these nuclei project to the cortex and it is activity within these cortico-thalamic loops which generates the rhythmic electrical activity of the EEG. Without this drive, the cortico-thalamic loops no longer function and conscious experience is absent. So it is not possible to have a small piece of the brain which is monitoring the environment and producing the conscious experiences which are reported.

A recent case in the AWARE study, reported by Dr Sam Parnia [21] is one of the few examples of a cardiac arrest and out of body experience occurring under close medical supervision in a prospective study.

The case concerns a middle aged man with diabetes who suffered a heart attack while at work. He was unaware of the seriousness of the episode but his colleagues called an ambulance and he was taken to hospital. The examining physician recognised that he was having a heart attack due to an occluded coronary artery and he was sent to the cardiac catheter laboratory to have a stent inserted. He was on the operating table and had drapes over his body placed in such a way that he was unable to see the procedures that were being carried out in his groin. He reports someone pressing in his groin, which is the standard practice with the injection of an anaesthetic and insertion of a catheter. The patient reports that he then became aware that a very beautiful woman (he later described her as an angel) up in the corner of the room in front of him, beckoning to him. The next thing he knew was that he was up on the ceiling reviewing the resuscitation process. Although he does not note any change in consciousness it was just before this time that his heart went into ventricular fibrillation , indicating that it had functionally stopped . He was in cardiac arrest. The team in the catheter lab immediately brought in an AED (automatic external defibrillator) of the type found in public places. They put the electrodes of this machine onto the patient and the machine then measured his cardiac activity, recognised that he was in ventricular fibrillation and gave the auditory command, Suggest Shock.

The shock was then given but failed to start the heart. When using this machine it is common practice if the shock fails to carry out a round of cardiac pulmonary stimulation (CPS). This was done and took two to three minutes. The machine then reanalysed his cardiac rhythm, noted the continuing ventricular fibrillation and gave a second auditory command, Suggest Shock. This was then given and the patient's heart re-started. Throughout the whole period of the ventricular fibrillation the patient reported that he was conscious and on the ceiling, watching the resuscitation process and hearing both the auditory commands.

The entire arrest was monitored by the Cardiac Catheter team and the subjective details of the patient's experiences were recounted by the patient.. Examination of the whole episode showed there could be no doubt that it happened as reported. There is clear evidence that the patient was in ventricular fibrillation and was dead between 11 and 15 seconds after his heart stopped. The length of time that this continued can be calculated because of the type of stimulation used and the number of shocks given – three to five minutes. This case illustrates that consciousness – i.e. awareness of your body in space, seeing and viewing , communicating with spiritual beings – are all possible when there is no electrical brain function and the patient is dead.

There are only two reasonable explanations for these findings. The first is brain based and argues that even an electrically silent brain is capable of perception - for which there is no evidence. The second is that mind and brain are not synonymous. It would suggest that mind and brain are so closely coupled before the heart stops, that it is difficult to see a difference between them. However, when brain function ceases, then mind appears no longer to be linked to brain function. For a full review of this possibility see Rousseau [22].

The similarity between the phenomena described in the cardiac arrest data and our research of ELEs, suggests that they may form a continuum. Dead relatives communicating with the person are common to both, as are the experiences of light and transcendent love. Taking a purely phenomenological view of the two sets of experiences, then the new model of dying would be that at the end-of-life wider experiences become more common and the dying person more open to them. It is sometimes suggested that a sudden death may deprive families and victims of the comfort of an ELE. This highlights the need to prepare for death while healthy – so that however suddenly it occurs, we are prepared to 'die right.'

'Dying Right'

"Although all of us will die, hardly anyone is prepared, or is preparing, to die right" [23]. The problem, according to Imhof, is that death is not taught as a medical subject, and 'dying right' is not part of medical studies and discussion of death, and the dying process, is rarely addressed in our Western culture.

The need now is to help palliative care workers to a better understanding of the dying process, and to bring back the idea of pastoral care and help to those who may not be religious, need to unburden themselves, but do not know how to do so. Our role as researchers, carers and educators is to give the medical and nursing professions permission to acknowledge and include all that we have discussed in their models of care. It can also mean helping patients in self-discovery and personal development as they approach death, perhaps by finding ways to express themselves through art, writing, poetry, music etc. Some of these activities have been reported to be the very spiritual work that people suddenly want to do as they realise they are approaching death. Many carers are increasingly aware of finding themselves in the role of the 'new priests at the bedside' –helping the dying they care for prepare for a good death. Patients who have firm religious beliefs or who have had the experience of visions etc often find their own reassurance in the face of death. But professional carers have the tools to help every dying patient, humanists, 'materialists' and nihilists alike, enrich, empower and heal their own lives and relationships as they prepare for the end of a life lived. The end-of-life experiences help provide a forum around which some of this discourse can take place.

The real barriers to a good death are those of unfinished business, such as unresolved emotions of guilt or hate, and the most effective tool in helping them is reconciliation. If we can help our patients recognise, and deal with, unfinished business, unresolved personal issues and family conflicts, we are ensuring as far as we can that they will experience a peaceful and 'good death'. Now is the time also to teach our patients about ELEs so that when they happen they can be prepared for the next step.

> "Suddenly she looked up at the window and seemed to stare intently up at it... ....She suddenly turned to me and said "Please Pauline, don't ever be afraid of dying. I have seen a beautiful light and I was going towards it.... it was so peaceful I really had to fight to come back." The next day when it was time for me to go home I said "Bye mum, see you tomorrow." She looked straight at me and said "I'm not worried about tomorrow and you mustn't be, promise me." Sadly she died the next morning....but I knew she had seen something that day which gave her comfort and peace when she knew she had only hours to live."

Dr. Christine Puchalski, Founder and Director of the George Washington Institute for Spiritual Health gives this very wise advice to those caring for the dying [24].

> "The key element of the spiritual history is listening to what is important to the patient and being truly present for the patient. This is at the root of compassionate caregiving."

REFERENCES

[1] Seravalli, E. 'The Dying Patient, the Physician and the Fear of Death'. *New England Journal of Medicine*, 1988. Dec. 1728-30.

[2] Kubler Ross, Elizabeth, 'What's it Like to be Dying'. *American Journal of Nursing,* 1971. 71, 1, 54-62. 1971

[3] Heyse-Morse, LH. 'On Spiritual Pain of Dying'. *Mortality*. 1996. 1, 3, 297-315.

[4] Steinhauser, K; Christakis, N; Clipp, E; McNeilly, M; McIntyre, L; Tulsky, J. "Factors Considered Important at the End-of-life by Patients, Family, Physicians, and Other Care Providers," *JAMA,* 2000. 284, 2476-2482

[5] Brayne, S; Farnham, C; Fenwick, P. An Understanding of the Occurrence of Deathbed Phenomena and its Effect on Palliative Care Clinicians. *American Journal of Hospice and Palliative Care*. 2006. 23, 1, 17-24

[6] Fenwick, P; Lovelace, H; Brayne, S. Comfort for the Dying. 5 year Retrospective and one year Prospective Studies of End-of-life Experiences. *Arch.Gerontol. Geriat.* 2010. 51(2), 173-9.

[7] Osis, K; Haraldsson, E. Deathbed Observations by Physicians and Nurses: A Cross-Cultural Survey. *The Journal for the American Society for Psychical Research*. 1977. 71, No 3.

[8] McConville, U. Ways of Knowing: Accounts of 'Sense of Presence' Experiences and Deathbed Visions 1969-1999. *Masters in Death & Society*, University of Reading. 2000.

[9] Fenwick, P; Fenwick, E. *The Art of Dying*. Continuum. 2009.

[10] Fenwick, P; Brayne, S. End-of-life Experiences: Reaching out for Compassion, Communication, and Connection: Meaning of Deathbed Visions and Coincidences. *Am.J. Hosp. Pallliat. Care*, 2011. 28(1), 7-15.

[11] Nahm, M; Greyson, B; Kelly, EW; Haraldsson, E. Terminal lucidity: a review and a case collection. *Arch Gerontol Geriatr.,* 2012 Jul-Aug, 55(1); 138-42.

[12] Byrd, RC. Positive therapeutic effects of intercessory prayer in a coronary care unit population. *Southern Medical Journal,* 1988. 81, 826-829.

[13] Sheldrake, R; Smart, P. Testing for telepathy in connection with e-mails. *Percept Mot Skills*. 2005. 101(3), 771-86.

[14] Achterberg, J; Cooke, K; Richards, T; Standish, L; Kozak, L; Lake, J. Evidence for Correlations between Distant Intentionality and Brain Function in Recipients: A Functional Magnetic Resonance Imaging Analysis. *Journal of Alternative and Complementary Medicine,* 2005. 11 (6).

[15] Parnia, S; Waller, D; Yeates, R; Fenwick, P. A qualitative and quantitative study of the incidence, features and aetiology of near death

experiences in cardiac arrest survivors. *Resuscitation*, 2001. 48, 149 – 156.

[16] Van Lommel, P; Wees Van, R; Meyers, V. Elfferich. Near-death experience in survivors of cardiac arrest: a prospective study in the 7. *Lancet*, 2001, 358, 2039-2045.

[17] Greyson, B. Incidence and Correlates of Near Death Experiences in a Cardiac Care Unit. *General Hospital Psychiatry*. 2003, 25, 269-276.

[18] Schwaninger, J. A prospective analysis of Near Death Experiences in cardiac arrest patients. *Journal of Near Death Experiences,* 2002, 20 (4).

[19] Sartori, P; Badham, P. *The Near Death Experience of Hospitalised Intensive Care Patients: a Five Year Clinical Study*. Edwin Mellen Press. Ltd. 2008.

[20] Holden, J; Greyson, B; James, D. *Handbook of Near-Death Experiences:30 years of investigation.* ABC-Clio. Ca. 2009.

[21] Parnia, S. *The Lazarus Effect . The Science that is Re-writing the Boundaries between Life and Death.* HarperOne. 2013.

[22] Rousseau, D. Mind, Souls and Nature: A Systems-Philosophical Analysis of the Mind-Body Relationship in the Light of Near Death Experiences. (Phd Thesis). University of Wales. *Trinity Saint David School of Theology*, Religious Studies and Islamic Studies. 2011.

[23] Imhof, AE. An Ars Moriendi for our Time: To Live a Fulfilled Life - to Die a Peaceful Death. http://userpage.fu-berlin.de/~aeimhof/ame.htm.

[24] Puchalski, C; Romer, L. Taking a Spiritual History allows Clinicians to Understand Patients more Fully. *Journal of Palliative Medicine,* 2000, 3(1), 129-137.

In: End-of-Life Care
Editors: Maria Rossi and Luiz Ortiz
ISBN: 978-1-62808-555-6

Chapter 3

DIABETES AND END-OF-LIFE CARE: ETHICAL ISSUES, PRACTICES AND CHALLENGES

Trisha Dunning[*]

Chair in Nursing and Director Centre for Nursing and Allied Health Research Deakin University and Barwon Health, Geelong, Australia

ABSTRACT

Diabetes is the most significant chronic disease and the global prevalence is increasing. Diabetes is associated with debilitating long term complications and other comorbidities that cause high rates of morbidity and mortality. Keeping blood glucose and other metabolic parameters within an acceptable, personalised range is important to comfort and quality of life but can be challenging, especially during end-of-life care.

Guidelines can help clinicians make appropriate care decisions; however, there is little research about what constitutes best practice diabetes care at the end-of-life: existing recommendations and guidelines blend the best available evidence with consensus opinion. In addition, there are important ethical and methodological considerations concerning research involving vulnerable people at the end-of-life. Chapter 3 describes the ethical and methodological issues that needed to be considered when developing guidelines for managing diabetes at the end-

[*] Phone: 61 03 42153288. Fax: 61 03 4215 3288. E-mail: trisha.dunning@ barwonhealth.org.au.

of-life and the contribution interviews with dying people and their family carers made to developing a guiding philosophy and to person-centred guidelines.

Keywords: Diabetes, end-of-life, guidelines, ethics, vulnerability, philosophy

INTRODUCTION

Life expectancy has increased in the past 20 years but diabetes is still among the top ten leading causes of death globally, many due to cardiovascular disease (McEwen et al. 2006; IDF 2012) but may be uniquely different among countries, regions and cultures (Foody et al. 2013). Diabetes-related deaths are not usually rapid, unlike deaths associated with catastrophic diseases such as pneumonia; however, diabetes-associated cardiac death can be sudden and 'silent,' thus cardiovascular disease presents particular challenges for people with diabetes and health professionals. Cardiovascular disease may represent an immediate death threat but will probably lead to death in the future (Pollard 1992).

Research suggests many people with serious illnesses report inadequate symptom control, fragmented care, and inadequate communication with health professionals. Their family care givers report significant stress (Gardner and Faan 2012).

However, many people, including health professionals, find it difficult to discuss dying and the value of making proactive decisions about end-of-life care. Australian national guidelines recommend discussing end-of-life issues, including advanced planning, when the prognosis is less than 12 months (Clayton et al. 2007). It is important to document such discussions in the individual's medical record.

END-OF-LIFE CARE

End-of-life care changes from active treatment to palliative care where the focus is not necessarily on extending life but helping people accept death. However, the underlying disease, in this case diabetes, might still need to be treated to promote comfort and quality of life until the terminal stage (National Health and Medical Research Council (NHMRC) 2009).

Health professionals can help people with diabetes proactively plan for end-of-life care.

Palliative care is defined as:

An approach that improves the quality of life of patients and their families facing the problems associated with life-threatening illness, through prevention and relief of suffering by means of early identification and impeccable assessment and treatment of pain and other problems, physical, psychosocial and spiritual.

(World Health Organisation (WHO) 2009)

THE END-OF-LIFE PROCESS

The end-of-life process consists of a series of transitions (NHMRC 2009) or stages: stable, unstable, deteriorating and terminal and usually lasts ~ 6–12 months (Palliative Care Outcomes Collaborative (PCOC) 2008). These stages are not linear, especially in diabetes where episodes of stable/unstable metabolic control can occur over years before the individual enters the final deteriorating and terminal stages.

Thus, people with diabetes may have a long progression to terminal care during which their diabetes needs to be managed but where a palliative approach may be warranted; for example people with end stage renal disease and severe cardiovascular disease who are stable but have a life limiting prognosis could benefit from the opportunity to make decisions about their preferred way of dying and document an advance care plan (ACP) and/or advance care directive (ACD) and other relevant documentation such as treatment withdrawal and to finalise their will. ACPs also help family members and carers make appropriate care decisions when the time comes.

The ACP could describe:

- How the individual wants each stage managed.
- Treatment preferences including continuing or withdrawing treatment.
- The value they place on well being and functional ability.
- Cultural and religious needs.

It is preferable to document an ACP proactively and preferably during a stable diabetes period. However, it is difficult to determine an individual's prognosis and to decide when to begin discussing advance care planning and end-of-life care with people with diabetes.

Likewise, most current diabetes management guidelines do not encompass end-of-life issues. People with diabetes consult health professionals regularly; hence, these consultations represent opportunities for proactive care planning. Early discussion about end-of-life issues enable the individual and their carers to decide when resuscitation is not warranted, make or updating wills, designate power of attorney if relevant, and make funeral arrangements. These decisions could help mitigate health professional and carer stress.

Importantly, people's perspectives change over time, and in different situations; therefore, health professionals need to help the individual make the best possible decision in the moment, and understand that an ACP made several years before may not reflect the individual's wishes at a different time (Geri Pal 2010). Thus, it is important to regularly clarify whether people's values and wishes have changed.

The key diabetes end-of-life management considerations are shown in table 1. Type 1 and type 2 diabetes are pathophysiologically different, but generally require similar care. The most significant difference is the absolute lack of insulin in type 1 diabetes, which predisposes the individual to diabetic ketoacidosis if insulin is withheld; although insulin may no longer be necessary in the last hours of life.

End-of-life care focuses on maintaining comfort and quality of life, managing unpleasant symptoms such as pain to reduce the symptom burden and activating the Liverpool Care Pathway to avoid unnecessary treatment and achieve a dignified death when appropriate (Ellershaw et al. 2003; Dunning et al. 2012 a). Providing spiritual and psychological support to the individual and their family/carers is essential.

Implementing end-of-life care represents a transition from curative to palliative care and is as important as curative care. The seemingly simple transition to palliative care is highly complex and emotion-laden. Proactively planning for end-of-life care should be incorporated into usual diabetes care and complication screening processes (Dunning 2010) and can improve people with diabetes' quality of life as well as diabetes management.

Diabetes-Specific End-of-life Guidelines

Some diabetes-specific guidelines have been developed and complement general palliative care guidelines such as:

Table 1. Overview of diabetes management at the end-of-life based on Dunning et al. 2010 and Diabetes UK 2012

Diabetes management should be integrated into the overall diabetes and palliative care plans and should be a collaborative process among relevant diabetes and palliative care clinicians and other clinicians where relevant, and make provision for:	
1	Providing individualised personalised care that includes preparing an ACP, identifying cultural, religious and spiritual beliefs and customs that influence how palliative care, death and care of the body and family/carers after death should be managed.
2	Making provision for communicating with the individual and their family/carers and among health professionals throughout the palliative care journey.
3	Identifying and managing pre-existing diabetes and diabetes pre-existing complications that affect management decisions such as medicine choices when renal and liver disease are present and can contribute to pain and discomfort. In addition, corticosteroid-induced hypeglycaemia is common in palliative care situations, in people with pre-existing diabetes and those with diabetes risk factors and increase discomfort (Giovannucci et al. 2010; Gannon and Dando 2010).
4	Identifying individuals at risk of corticosteroid-induced diabetes when people are admitted to palliative care and/or when steroid medicines are prescribed, detecting diabetes early, and managing diabetes that develops following corticosteroid use (Dunning 1996; Du 2008).
5	Identifying risk of hypoglycaemia and developing strategies to reduce episodes of and manage hypoglycaemia. Hypoglycaemia can be individually or collectively related to GLMs, low hepatic glucose reserves, particularly if the individual is malnourished or has hepatic metastases, renal impairment or malabsorption due to gastrointestinal disturbance such autonomic neuropathy, anorexia and cachexia syndrome.
6	Choosing a safe, effective medicines and medicine regimen using quality use of medicine principles to achieve optimal glycaemic targets for the individual and the PCOC stage. Renal and hepatic function is often altered and gastrointestinal disturbance and impaired glucose absorption is common, which, along with the prognosis, and the individual's care decisions, influences medicine choices. Many oral GLM might be contraindicated and insulin might be a safer, simpler option but only consensus evidence is available for the latter recommendation (Dunning et al. 2010, Diabetes UK 2012, and Australian Diabetes Society (ADS) 2012).
7	Providing adequate nutrition and hydration on an individual basis depending on life expectancy and nutritional needs. People who are actively dying do not experience hunger largely due to the effects of starvation and consequent ketone production but they may experience thirst, which can be alleviated by mouth care (Kedziera 2001).

Table 1. (Continued)

8	Avoiding diabetes-related emergencies such as ketoacidosis, hyperosmolar states, lactic acidosis, and severe hypoglycaemia and pain and discomfort due to unnecessary hospital admissions.
9	Deciding when to withdraw treatment and activating the Liverpool Care Pathway when the individual is dying (Ellershaw et al. 2003).
10	Supporting spiritual growth. Spirituality is a broader concept than religion, although it might encompass religion. Spirituality refers to the transformational process of finding meaning and purpose in life and an inner sense of coherence and resilience (Parsian andDunning 2009). Spirituality enables people to positively cope with life stressors. Significantly, people can find meaning and purpose in life when they are dying. However, spirituality can be affected by grief and loss (Puchalski 2011). Spirituality also affects family/carers' ability to cope. The factors that give meaning and purpose to people's lives influences their end-of-life care decisions. Spirituality should be encompassed in the medical history and regularly evaluated including when there is a change in clinical status. Spiritual distress and depression can overlap and manifest as demoralisation, people can be depressed and have no hope or be depressed and feel isolated from God (Puchalski 2011). However, people can have spiritual distress without being depressed.

Palliative Care

- National Guideline for a Palliative Approach in Residential Aged Care (Australian Commonwealth Department Health and Aging 2006)
- National Health and Medical Research Council (2011) Ethical Framework for Integrating Palliative Care principles into the Management of Advanced terminal and Chronic Conditions.

Diabetes-Specific

- Dunning et al. (2010) Guidelines for Managing Diabetes at the end-of-life.
- End-of-life Care Strategy (Diabetes UK) and Scotland End-of-life care Strategy (2008).0.

The UK and Dunning et al.'s guidelines are largely consensus based due to the limited amount of research into the area and the ethical and methodological issues that arise when conducting research involving vulnerable people such as those who are dying.

Developing Diabetes-Specific Guidelines for End-of-life Care: The Process

Dunning et al. followed recommended guideline development processes (NHMRC 2005) to develop their guidelines, see figure 1, which provides an overview of the guideline development process.

Literature Review

As indicated an established, transparent systematic process was followed to identify and synthesise the best available evidence relating to diabetes and end-of-life care (Petticrew and Roberts 2006). The literature review yielded only 10 relevant publications despite searching a range of databases such as EMBASE and Medline via PubMed and using various MESH and MeSH search terms and combinations of terms such as diabetes, end-of-life, dying, and death. The reference lists of publications were hand searched to identify relevant publications not identified in the search.

In addition, the grey literature in APAIS (health) and book shops were searched and yielded several books and other publications that described people and carers' experience of death and dying. The outcomes of interest were:

- Systematic reviews or other publications that described care of people with diabetes at the end-of-life.
- People with diabetes' perspectives of end-of-life care and what it should encompass.
- General descriptions of end-of-life care that could be adapted to managing diabetes at the end-of-life.
- Family/carers' perspectives of managing their loved one's diabetes at the end-of-life.

Two researchers independently reviewed and rated the literature and then discussed their reviews.

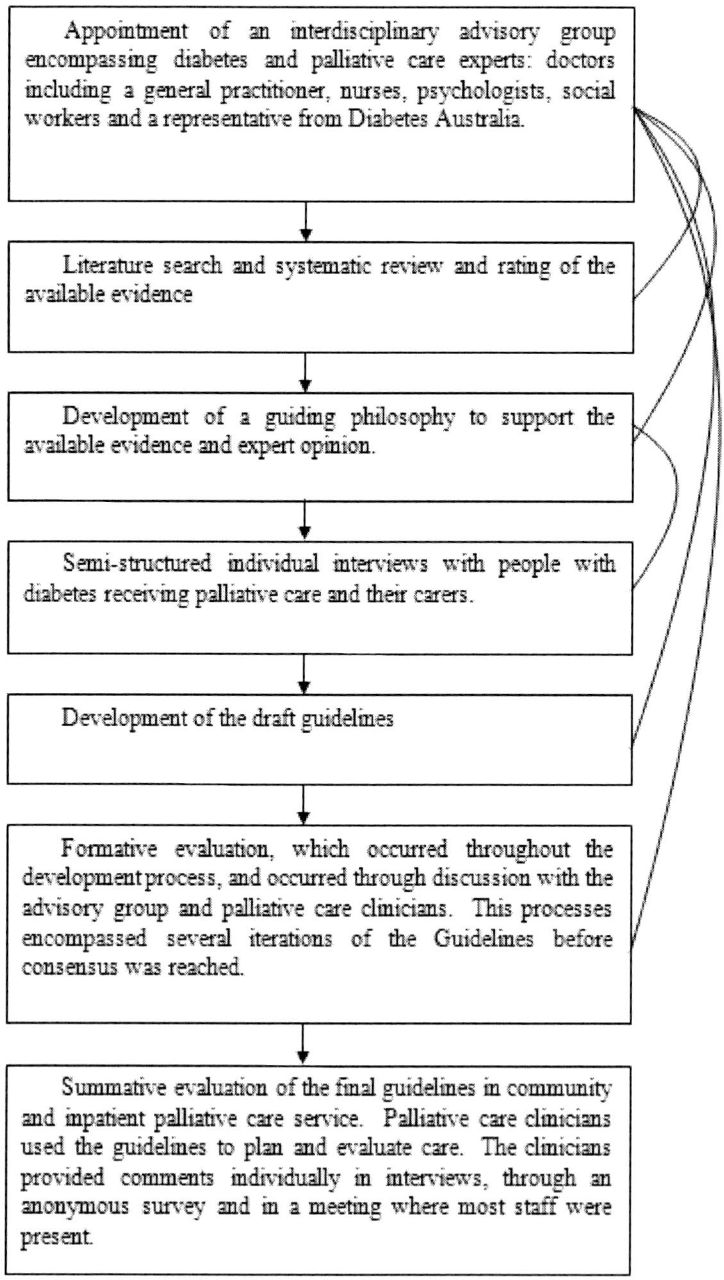

Figure 1. Overview of the six stage process Dunning et al. (2011 and 2012) used to develop guidelines for managing diabetes at the end-of-life.

Not unexpectedly, no randomised controlled trials or systematic reviews were identified. Ten relevant publications were identified that made care recommendations about diabetes end-of-life care life, however, the recommendations were not evidence-based and most recommendations were based on the recommendations in one paper. Several authors remarked on the need for diabetes-specific end-of-life management guidelines.

Some non-diabetes related literature provided useful information about people's general end-of-life care needs that are applicable to people with diabetes. These texts were reviewed using the Critical Appraisal Skills Programme qualitative studies tool (CASP) if they were qualitative studies. In addition, thematic analysis of the information in qualitative studies and books and articles in the grey literature were subject to thematic analysis using Ritchie and Spencer's Framework Method (Ritchie and Spencer 1994).

The qualitative literature suggests dying people expect health professionals to respect 'their ways of being' and understand time is precious at the end-of-life. They find waiting for appointments and test results distressing, and want some indication of 'how much time they have left' to enable them to put their affairs in order (Pesut et al. 2012).

People want health professionals to deliver care without being intrusive and to work with and support their family/carers. In addition, people want some general 'signposts' or cues to help them recognise when they are entering the deteriorating stage to enable them to make realistic decisions about dying (Pesut et al. 2012). Loss of privacy during the final dying process, especially in hospitals and hospices, but also at home, is a concern for some people.

People with diabetes and family/carers worry about their lack of knowledge and skills to undertake diabetes self-care when their loved ones can no longer self-care, worry about unnecessarily hastening death or causing distress and pain (Dunning et al. 2010). Likewise, carer participants in Pesut et al.'s (2012) study indicated health professionals often overestimate carers' knowledge, when in fact they 'do not know what questions to ask.' .Thus, educating family/carers and helping them ask pertinent questions is part of personalised care at the end-of-life.

Interviews with People with Diabetes and Carers

Dunning et al. conducted interviews with people with diabetes at the end-of-life (n = 14) and their families (n = 10) to determine how they wanted their diabetes managed to supplement the meagre 'evidence' (Savage et al. 2012). Interviews were considered to be more likely to yield in-depth information than questionnaires despite the vulnerability of the sampling population. An interview guide was developed and all questions were asked in each interview but not necessarily in the same order to enable the conversation to flow sensibly (Gilbert 2007). Active listening, using probing and clarifying questions during the interviews and constant comparative data analysis enabled the researchers to explore emerging issues as they arose and ensure data saturation was reached.

The interviews were challenging, emotionally demanding for the researchers and the participants but provided valuable information from key stakeholders, people with diabetes, about how they wanted their diabetes managed at the end-of-life, not previously documented. All interviews were conducted face-to-face and most were undertaken in peoples' homes (n = 14). These people were all receiving palliative care and were in various stages of the dying process: stable, unstable, and deteriorating (Palliative Care Outcomes Collaboration (PCOC) 2008). Family carers, mostly spouses (n = 10), were also interviewed separately from their relatives (Dunning et al. 2012 a and b; Savage et al. 2012).

Dunning et al. (2012 a) used the information derived from the interviews as well as from a thematic analysis of people's published stories about their dying experiences (personal narratives), the review of the available literature and quality use of medicines principles (QUM) (National Prescribing Service 2009) to develop a guiding philosophy or conceptual framework for their guidelines.

GUIDING PHILOSOPHY

The other difference from usual guideline development processes was developing a guiding philosophy to ensure the final guidelines were consistent with palliative and diabetes care philosophies, encompassed individualised person-centred care and followed ethical principles. The philosophy was developed using an iterative process through discussions with the Guideline reference group and palliative care clinicians.

Thus, the guideline development process differed from usual guideline development processes, in that some of the 'experts' consulted were people with diabetes. Interviewing the intended care recipients is consistent with current recommendations for patient engagement and patient-centred care, although it is not an established aspect of guideline development processes.

Significantly, the interviews yielded important information about people with diabetes feelings about controlling blood glucose levels to promote comfort and quality of life and the fact that people with diabetes did not regard blood glucose monitoring as painful or intrusive, rather, they felt it yielded important information on which to base care decisions. In addition, it was a familiar routine in a changing life phase. Likewise, people with diabetes felt continuing glucose lowering medicines until the terminal stage helped control symptoms, rather than prolong life (Savage et al. 2012). These views are different from the views of many health professionals (Quinn et al. 2006) but helped define the standard of end-of-life care people with diabetes expect from health professionals.

Ethical Issues

The decision to conduct interviews with vulnerable dying people to complement the available evidence raised ethical and methodological issues that needed to be addressed. Similar ethical issues also emerge when providing care for dying people.

The core ethical principles date from ancient times and are enshrined in the Hippocratic Oath and the Florence Nightingale Pledge as well as the Declaration of Geneva (1948); International Code of Ethics (1959/1988) and the ethics statements of various research and professional organisations. These statements were derived from values, principles and standards and duty of care owed to people receiving care. The principles are beneficence, non-maleficence, autonomy, Justice, Informed consent, privacy and vulnerability.

Beneficence

From a clinical care perspective beneficence involves ensuring care benefits the individual and health professionals act in the best interest of the individual.

People often view the issue as a choice between aggressive treatment to save or extend life and accepting death as a natural part of life and providing care to promote comfort and quality of life for whatever time is left (RAND Health 2006), both are equally valuable aspects of care. Health professionals and carers are often confronted with their own mortality or that of a loved one, which can compromise their ability to be objective and their decisions about what constitutes the best interests of the individual. Likewise, people with diabetes could interpret the focus on palliative care as 'giving up on them' and losing control over their diabetes-related care decisions.

The individual must have enough information to actively participate in discussion about whether it is appropriate to continue treatment and to weigh the benefits, risks and physical, mental and spiritual burden involved in the care options (Murray et al. 2004). A combination of usual diabetes care and a palliative approach might benefit some people with diabetes and cardiovascular disease and/or renal disease. Controlling hyperglycaemia is essential to comfort, symptom control and quality of life.

Decisions about treatment benefit require appropriate discussion about risks and benefits and appropriate use of treatment with the individual concerned in the appropriate language and individualised to their situation. Many treatments produce significant side effects and discomfort and confer little long term benefit. In addition aggressive treatment is associated with a high risk of depression in bereaved caregivers (Steinhauser et al. 2000; Mack et al. 2012). Beneficence related to participating in research also needed to be considered when applying for ethics approval to interview people with diabetes at the end-of-life when developing the guidelines. Some researchers interpret beneficence as benefiting research in general and not necessarily the individual participants (Ford and Reulter 1990) but the value/benefit of research is often questioned when small samples are involved, as was the case with Dunning et al.'s guideline interviews. Likewise, the interviews had the potential to cause considerable distress and represented an additional burden to potential participants, hence strategies need to be in place to minimise such risks. In addition the risks need to be clearly explained to potential participants before they consent to participate.

Non-Maleficence

Non-maleficence is embodied in the statement: *primun non nocere* 'first do no harm.' It is almost impossible to guarantee no harm will result. Acting in the best interests of the individual and discussing the relevant issues openly and honestly will likely help reduce harm in clinical care and research. Appropriate documentation is also essential for example ACP and ACD and other relevant documents.

Autonomy

Personal autonomy and respect for people, which is consistent with the concept of self-determination, is a key aspect of informed consent. People have a right to refuse medical treatment; they also have a responsibility to make their wishes known.

These rights and responsibilities assume people have the capacity to make informed decisions without coercion. Autonomy applies equally to clinical care and research. As indicated, people can indicate their care preferences when their decision-making capacity is intact by documenting their wishes in ACPs and ACDs.

Autonomy is closely linked to independence and dignity and is embodied in ancient Greek philosophy of autarky (Audi 1999). Loss of independence does not automatically imply decision-making autonomy is lost. Significantly, relationships in some cultures that involve mutual obligations; for example, Australian Aboriginal peoples and Chinese peoples' philosophy of filial piety might imply a different perspective of autonomy and the rights of the individual with respect to the collective right of the community.

Justice

There are various kinds of justice. For example distributive justice, which is concerned with equitable allocation of medical resources (Walker 2012) can arise when the cost of treatment is high and when resources are scarce, for example kidneys for people on the transplant list. Justice-related issues can affect individuals, carers and health professionals. Justice can be infringed if cultural issues are not considered.

Justice is served if under and over treatment are avoided and the individual receives the 'right' treatment for their current needs. A justice-related issue emerged in Dunning et al.'s guideline research when staff acted as 'gatekeepers' and made decisions about the individual's interest in participating in the interviews and whether participating was in their best interest without discussing the issue with the individuals involved. Such decisions were made from the health professional's perspective of the 'best interest of the individual' but deprived people of the opportunity of contributing valuable information and hindered recruitment.

The recruitment process was amended with ethics approval and the researchers were able to contact potential participants after staff gave them an information pack about the study. People volunteered to participate, even in the last stages of life and informed other people at the end-of-life in their networks about the study, which indicated they wanted to contribute to the study. Thus, an expected consequence was snowball sampling. 'Gatekeeping' might have compromised people's autonomy and ability to give informed consent.

Informed Consent

Informed consent helps protect people's right to autonomy and personal veracity. In order to provide informed consent, people must have the relevant information in a format and language they can understand about what the study involves, what they will be expected to do, as well as be given time to consider the invitation to participate. Informed consent is also essential in clinical care and is predicated on good communication and accurate documentation.

Privacy

People have a right to privacy, yet technology enables people's right to privacy to be infringed without them knowing and without their consent. Dunning et al. had access to very private information through conducting the interviews in people's homes/personal spaces (participant preference), they would not normally have access to. Likewise the sample size was small; deidentifying information, using codes and only reporting group information might not protect people's privacy in small samples. People were informed that the way they used language and words ('voice') could identify them even when data were deidentified.

Vulnerability

Vulnerability is defined in different ways and is likely to differ among the various PCOC stages and other life stages and events. Vulnerability can be cumulative and have a cascading effect on what, where and how care is delivered. For example, a vulnerable individual might be admitted to hospital instead of receiving palliative care at home. However, having their family member in hospital may actually reduce family/carers sense of vulnerability because they have access to trained staff.

Vulnerability itself does not exclude people from participating in research or making care decisions provided they are able to give informed consent. Vulnerability can be a manifestation of illness or disability (Chochinov and Steinstra 2012) that can affect people's ability to make informed decisions. However, the focus on physical vulnerability does not address key issues such as what is 'normal.' Gill (2006) argued that people with disabilities are not necessarily innately vulnerable but can be made to feel vulnerable by society and health professionals' assumptions about their capacity (imposed vulnerability).

Imposed vulnerability emerged in Dunning et al.'s (2012 b) interviews when staff made assumptions about people's capacity to participate in interviews. Imposed vulnerability could mean people are offered fewer options including the option to participate in research.

Kipnis (2001) divided vulnerability into five bioethical domains. Dunning et al. found Kipnis' domains valuable when designing the interviews for the Guideline study.

People who participated in Dunning et al.'s study were a highly vulnerable, individually and collectively, in four of the five domains Kipnis described. Institutional vulnerability was reduced in Dunning et al.'s study because most people choose to be interviewed in their own homes; however, that introduced another form of vulnerability and, as discussed, raised privacy issues.

METHODOLOGICAL ISSUES

Dunning et al. decided to use a qualitative research method, individual interviews, to enhance existing evidence about end-of-life care knowing qualitative research is not considered to be high level evidence but believing it was the best method to address the study aim and achieve methodological integrity. Dunning et al. were careful to ensure they maintained rigor in the study.

Methodological issues were:

- The sample was recruited from a vulnerable group who were making decisions about their care and confronting the end of their life. Thus, the burden of participation needed to be considered.

- The nature of qualitative research and ensuring rigor was maintained by researcher reflexivity, interviewing skills, compiling field notes and reflecting on professional boundaries and the different roles of nurse and researcher, and the need to be able to debrief after each interview
- The process of accessing and recruiting potential participants. Palliative care staff was very protective of the people they were caring for and in many cases decided the individual would not want to participate or was too ill to participate without consulting the individual. While staff concern for the patient's wellbeing is laudable, it did not conform to the ethical principle, justice, and people's right to be heard.

CONCLUSION

Combining interviews with a literature review and using a guiding philosophy to develop guidelines for managing diabetes at the end-of-life ensured people with diabetes' and family/carers' perspectives were understood, which helped ensure the final guidelines were person-centred. Vulnerability emerged as a key ethical issue when designing the study, applying for ethics approval and conducting the study.

Vulnerability should not automatically exclude people from participating in research but they must be able to give informed consent and be given enough information to make an informed, autonomous decision about participating.

'Good' diabetes care may require a palliative approach in the last year of life as well as continuing usual diabetes management strategies and individualising metabolic targets. The interviews in the current study show people with diabetes want their blood glucose controlled and blood glucose monitoring continued to promote comfort, safety and quality of life. People with diabetes should be encouraged to proactively document their end-of-life care needs rather than leaving such decision to the last stages when decision-making capacity might be impaired.

Dunning et al.'s Guidelines can be accessed on Error! Hyperlink reference not valid. The Guidelines are endorsed by the Australian Diabetes Educators Association and the Department of Health Palliative Care Clinical network Victoria until 2015 when they will be revised.

REFERENCES

Australian Diabetes Society (ADS) (2012) Guideline for routine glucose control in hospital ADS, Canberra.

Australian Government Department of Health and Ageing. (2006). National guidelines for a palliative approach to residential aged care. Enhanced version. Church lands: Edith Cowan University.

Audi R. (1999). The Cambridge Dictionary of Philosophy. Cambridge University Press (p 62).

Critical appraisal Skills Programme (CASP) for qualitative studies www.phm.nhs.uk/Pages/PHD/CAP.htm (accessed January 2013).

Chochinov H, Steinstra D. (2012) Vulnerability and palliative care. P*alliative and Supportive Care* 10:1–2.

Clayton J, Hancock K. Butow P, Tattersall M, Currow D. (2007) Clinical practice guidelines for communicating prognosis and end-of-life issues with adults in the advanced stages of life limiting illness and their caregivers. *Medical Journal of Australia* 186 (12): 77–86.

Department of Health Palliative Care Clinical Network Victoria www.health.vic.gov.au/clinicalnetwork/publications.htm (accessed February 2013).

Diabetes UK (2012) End-of-life diabetes care; a strategy document commissioned by Diabetes UK, Diabetes UL London.

Du L. (2008) Management of steroid-induced diabetes in patients with COPD. *Medscape Diabetes and Endocrinology* http://www.medscape.com/viewarticle/458619 (accessed October 2012).

Dunning, T. (1996). Corticosteroid medications and diabetes mellitus. *Practical Diabetes International, 13*(6), 186-188.

Dunning T, Savage S, Duggan N, Martin P. (2010) Guidelines for Managing Diabetes at the End-of-life available from http:// clearing house.adma.org.au/browse-resources/guideline/guidelines-for-managing-diabetes-at-the-end-of-life/details.html.

Dunning T, Savage S, Duggan N, Martin P. (2012 a) developing clinical guidelines for end-of-life care: blending evidence and consensus. *International Journal of Palliative Nursing* 18 (8):397–405.

Dunning T, Savage S, Duggan N, Martin P. (2012 b) Diabetes and end-of-life: ethical and methodological issues in gathering evidence. *Scandinavian Journal Caring Sciences* doi: 10.111/j.1471.612.2012.01016.x.

Ellershaw, J. (2003). Introduction. In J. Ellershaw and S. Wilkinson (Eds.), Care of the dying. A pathway to excellence. Oxford: Oxford University Press.

Ford L, Reuter L (1990 Ethical dilemmas associated with small samples. *Journal of Advanced Nursing* 15:187–191.

Foody J, Huo Y, Ji L, Zhao D, Boyd D, Meng H, Shiff S, Hu D. (2003)Unique and varied contributions of traditional CVD risk factors: a systematic literature review of CAD risk factors in China. *Clinical Medicine Insights* 7:59–86.

Gannon C, Dando N. (2010) Dose-sensitive steroid-induced hyperglycaemia. *Palliative Medicine* 24 **7:**737–739.

Gardner D, Faan F. (2012) Quality in life and death: can we have conversations? *Nurse Economist* 30 (4):224–226.

GeriPal (2010) Advanced care planning: accounting for changing perspectives. http://www.thecamreport.com2010/09/advanced-care-planning-accounting-for-changing-perspectives (accessed August 2012).

Gill C. (2006) Disability, constructed vulnerability and socially conscious palliative care. *Journal of Palliative Care* 22:183–191.

Gilbert N. (2008) Researching Social Life London, Sage.

Giovannucci E, Harlan D, Archer M, Bergenstal R, Gapstur S, Habel L, Pollak M, Regensteiner J, Yee D. (2010) *Diabetes and Cancer Diabetes Care* 7: 1674–1685.

International Diabetes Federation (IDF) (2012) Diabetes Atlas Brussels, IDF.

Kedziera P. (201) hydration, thirst and nutrition in Farrell B, Coyle N (eds) Textbook of Palliative Nursing, New York Oxford University Press.

Kipnis K. (2001) Vulnerability in research subjects: a bioethical taxonomy in Ethical and Policy Issues in Research Involving Human Research Participants, National Bioethics Advisory Commission, Bethesda, Maryland, USA.

Mack J, Cronin A, Keating N, Taback N, Huskamp A, Malin J, Earle C, Weeks J. (2012) Associations between end-of-life discussion charactristics and care received near death: a prospective cohort study. *Journal of Clinical Oncology* 10.1200/JCo.012.42.6055.

McEwen L, Kim C, Haan M, Ghosh M, Lantz P. (2006) Diabetes reporting as cause of death: results from the Translating Resaerch into Action for Diabetes (TRIAD) study, *Diabetes Care*: 29 2):147–253).

Murray M, Miller T, Fiset V, O'Connor A, Jacobsen M. (2001) Decision support: helping patients and families find balance at the end of life.. *International Journal of Palliative Nursing* 10 (6):270 - 277.

National Health and Medical Research Council. (2005). A guide to the development, implementation and evaluation of clinical practice guidelines. Canberra: National Health and Medical Research Council.

NHMRC (2009) Ethical issues involved in the transitions to palliation and end-of-life care for people with chronic conditions: A discussion paper for patients, carers and health professionals. Canberra, NHMRC.

National Prescribing Service Ltd and Palliative Care Australia. (2009). Achieving quality use of medicines in the community for palliative and end-of-life care: A consultation report. Sydney: National Prescribing Service Ltd.

Palliative Care Outcomes Collaboration (PCOC) (2008): PCOC Assessment tool definitions: Phase V 1.2.

Parsian N, Dunning T. (2009) Spirituality and coping in young adults with diabetes: a cross sectional study. *European Diabetes Nursing* 6L100-104.

Petticrew M, Roberts H (2006) Systematic Reviews in the Social Sciences: A practical guide. Oxford: Blackwell Publishing.

Pesut B, McLeod B, Hole R, Dalhuisen M. (2012) Rural nursing and quality end-of-life care: palliative care, palliative approach or somewhere in between *Advances in Nursing Science* 35 **4:**288–304.

Pollard B. (1992) Palliative care—is it the answer? Error! Hyperlink reference not valid. (accessed December 2012).

Puchalski C. (2011) Spirituality is an important component of patient care. *Web*MD Professional http://www.medscape.com/viewarticle/738237 (accessed August 2012).

Quinn, K., Hudson, P., and Dunning, T. (2006). Diabetes management in patients receiving palliative care. *Journal of Pain and Symptom Management, 32*(3), 275–286.

RAND Health (2006) Refining and reframing health care for the last years of life. www.rand.org/pub/research_briefs/RB9178/index/html (accessed February 2013).

Ritchie Spencer (1994) Qualitative data analysis for applied policy research. In A. Bryman and R. Burgess (Eds.), Analysing qualitative data (pp. 173–194). London: Routledge.

Savage S, Dunning T, Duggan N, Martin P. (2012) The experiences and care preferences of people with diabetes at the end-of-life: a qualitative study *Journal of Hospice and Palliative Nursing* 14 (4): 293–302.

Steinhauser K E, Christakis N A, Clipp E C, McNeilly M, McIntyre L, Tulsky J A. (2000). Factors considered important at the end-of-life by individuals, family, physicians and other care providers. *Journal American Medical Association* 284: (19) 2476–2482.

Temel J, Greer J, Gallagher E, Jackson V, Lennes I, Muzikansky A, Park E, Pirl W. (2012) Electronic prompt to improve patent outpatient code status documentation for patients with advanced lung cancer *Journal of Clinical Oncology* D doi: 10.1200/jco.2012.43.2203 (accessed February 2013).

Walker R. 9 (2012) Ethical issues in end-of-life care. Lee Moffitt Cancer Center and Research Institute Error! Hyperlink reference not valid. (accessed February 2013).

World Health Organisation (WHO) (2009) Definition of Palliative Care www.who.int/cancer/palliative/definition/en (accessed December 2012).

In: End-of-Life Care
Editors: Maria Rossi and Luiz Ortiz
ISBN: 978-1-62808-555-6

Chapter 4

AFTER THE DEATH OF A LOVED ONE: HELPING FAMILIES TO COPE

Beatriz Gil-Juliá[*] and Rafael Ballester-Arnal
Facultad de Ciencias de la Salud,
Universitat Jaume I de Castellón, Spain

ABSTRACT

The End-of-Life Care requires a global and holistic approach to provide an excellent care, meeting the needs of both, the person who is dying and their relatives.

In this sense, it is important to recognize that the family, including close friends and carers, has a vital role during this process. They need to be closely involved in their loved one care as well as they have their own needs, which are not only present before and during death but also after the person's death.

Good end of life care does not stop at the point of death, and the proper emotional support is required by family members and friends to cope with their loss.

After the loss of a loved person, -one of the most stressful and painful events that people experience in their lives-, bereavement appears as a natural response. Most of people come to terms with this universal experience without requiring specialized psychotherapy. However, for a significant minority of bereaved people who struggle deeply and for a

[*] Corresponding author: Email: bgil@uji.es.

prolonged period of time, grief is complicated. In those circumstances we would be talking about complicated grief or prolonged grief disorder (Boelen & Prigerson, 2007; Neimeyer, 2008; Prigerson et al., 1995; Shear et al., 2011). The aim of this chapter is to revise the main issues related to grief and bereavement, including the definition of these terms, stages and tasks of grief, the description of the different types of grief reactions, complicated grief and treatments for helping bereaved people.

INTRODUCTION

The loss of a loved one can be considered one of the most stressful and painful events that people experience in their lives. It is an experience that occurs sooner or later in nearly everyone's life.

In the wake of loss, what do we understand by grief, mourning and bereavement? Are they synonymous terms? Although sometimes they are used interchangeably they differ, however, in their clinical manifestations. *Grief* has been defined as the process of physical, psychological and social reactions to the perception of loss. *Mourning* is the cultural response to grief, and like other reactions is socially and culturally influenced. Finally, *bereavement* is the state of having suffered the loss of someone close through death (Rando, 1984). In this sense, bereavement is a universal experience to which most people tend to adjust properly. It is experienced, as a natural response to loved one's death, along with suffering and distress. Nevertheless, for a significant minority of bereaved people grief can be complicated, struggling deeply and for a prolonged period of time. In those circumstances the need for treatment should be considered, especially if we take into account that bereavement is a severe stressor that can trigger the onset of a physical or mental disorder as well as can worsen previous pathologies (Shear et al., 2011).

Health professionals need to recognize when the grief process is normal and when they would be talking about complicated grief or prolonged grief disorder (Boelen & Prigerson, 2007; Neimeyer, 2008; Prigerson et al., 1995; Shear et al., 2011).

STAGES AND TASKS OF GRIEF

Throughout years, the general notion in response to loss is that people advance through a series of stages in the grieving process. Relevant authors in this field as Bowlby (1961) and Parkes (1972) proposed a stage theory of grief including four stages (shock-numbness, yearning-searching, disorganization-despair, and reorganization). Likewise, Kübler-Ross (1969), adapted Bowlby and Parkes' theory to describe five stages to go through by terminally ill patients attempting to cope with their own impeding death (denial-isolation, anger, bargaining, depression, and acceptance).

Not many attempts have been made to explicitly test the stage theory of grief. The most important of these attempts was conducted by Maciejewski, Zhang, Block, and Prigerson (2007), who found normal patterns of grief processing over time following the natural death of a loved one. However, these findings raised some controversy, and opposing opinions regarding the stage theory of grief were swift (Bonanno & Boerner, 2007; Silver & Wortman, 2007). Later, another study was carried out by Holland and Neimeyer (2010) aimed to provide a conceptual replication and extension of Maciejewski and colleagues' findings in a sample of young adults who had been bereaved by natural and violent causes. These authors found limited support for stage theory.

Despite this open controversy, it is not infrequent to hear about the importance of the stage theory. What might explain this? In Prigerson and Maciejewski words (2008), "it may reflect a desire to make sense of how the mind comes to accept events and circumstances that it finds wholly unacceptable" (pp. 435).

Many researchers of grief and bereavement process have proposed stages of normal grief (Bowlby, 1980; Engel, 1964; Glick, Weiss & Parkes, 1974; Lindemann, 1944; Parkes, 1972; Shuchter & Zisook, 1993). Nevertheless, we need to be cautioned. These stages would be useful insofar as they show a global landscape for grieving people as general guidelines but do not command necessarily where the bereaved has to be in the grieving process. At this point it is worth noting, in line with Kübler-Ross (1969) and as Shuchter and Zisook stated in 1993 that "Grief is not a linear process with concrete boundaries but, rather, a composite of overlapping fluid phases that vary from person to person" (pp. 23). It is of great importance bearing in mind the individual variability, considering both, the many kinds of emotions we can experience after a loss and the order in which we experience them. There is no grieving process like to another.

Instead of stages, other authors considered more appropriate to talk about "tasks" in the grieving process (Worden, 1982, 1997; Worden & Winokuer, 2011), since they imply that the person is an active element in the process, while phases could denote certain passivity. These authors defined four tasks of mourning: (1) to acknowledge the reality of the loss, (2) to process the pain of grief, (3) to adjust to a world without the deceased (4) to find an enduring connection with the deceased in the midst of embarking on a new life.

Similarly, Parkes and Weiss (1983) considered necessary three tasks for recovery from grief: (1) intellectual recognition and explanation of the loss, (2) emotional acceptance of the loss and (3) the assumption of a new identity.

At this regard it is important to assume as Worden and Winokuer state that "tasks are not linear and people go back and forth between them as they adapt to the loss" (pp. 64).

Grief Reactions

After the death of a loved one people experience a wide variety of physical, emotional, cognitive, social and behavioral disruptions.

Grief reactions may be similar to those observed in some physical or mental disorders. In fact, different studies have revealed that important proportions of bereaved individuals even meet criteria for disorders such as major depression (Zisook, Shuchter, Sledge, Paulus, & Judd, 1994), post-traumatic stress-disorder (PTSD) (Schut, De Keijser, Van den Bout, & Dijkhuis, 1991) and other anxiety disorders (Jacobs et al., 1990).

It is important to be careful in the interpretation of certain expressions of grief that may appear as pathological when they actually are natural and appropriate manifestations, given the circumstances of the loss.

Below, the main reactions to grief are shown (Lacasta & Soler, 2004; Latiegi, 1999; Worden, 1982), considering that they could vary from person to person as well as not all of them are experienced by all bereaved individuals.

- Feelings: sadness, anxiety, apathy, loss of interest in usual activities annoyance, anger, guilt, loneliness, abandonment, helplessness, numbness, strangeness with respect to himself/herself and to the global world.
- Cognitions: disbelief, confusion, worry, ruminations, flashbacks and intrusive thoughts, sense of presence, visual and/or auditory hallucinations, difficulties with attention, concentration and memory, cognitive distortions.
- Physical sensations: empty in the stomach and/or dry mouth, tightness in chest/throat, shortness of breath and/or palpitations,

hypersensitivity to noise, sense of depersonalization, lack of energy/weakness.

- Behaviors: sleep and/or feeding disturbances, distracted behavior, social isolation, cry and/or sigh, carry or hoard objects, visit places familiar to the deceased, call and/or talk to the deceased, hyper-hypo activity, avoid reminders of the deceased.

Despite such an emotional roller coaster, it is noteworthy that grief is not only related to pain. According to Zisook and Shear (2009) in an uncomplicated grief process, painful experiences go hand in hand with positive feelings (e.g., relief, joy, peace, and happiness). Nonetheless, frequently these positive feelings cause negative emotions of disloyalty and guilt in the bereaved. Likewise, these authors highlight that at least one investigation (Bonanno, Wortman & Nesse, 2004) has found that positive feelings at 6 months following a death are a sign of resilience and associated with good long-term outcomes.

Table 1. Stages of the grieving process

Lindemann	Parkes &Bowlby	Engel	Kübler-Ross
Shock and disbelief	Numbness	Shock and disbelief	Denial and isolation
Acute mourning	Yearning and searching	Developing awareness	Anger
Resolution	Disorganization and despair	Restitution	Bargaining
	Reorganization	Resolving the loss	Depression
		Idealization	Acceptance
		The outcome	

COMPLICATED GRIEF

Most bereaved individuals adjust fairly well to the death of a loved one, though this "uncomplicated" process entails suffering. Usually, they feel very sad and distressed, and miss their loved one, sometimes terribly.

What does it make the difference between complicated and uncomplicated grief? Prigerson (2004) reveals that "the important distinction between complicated and uncomplicated grief is that in the latter instance, the survivors are able to move on with their lives and pave a new way for themselves" (pp. 38). And this is possible for 80-90% of bereaved individuals. Unfortunately, 10-20% of bereaved people experience Complicated Grief (CG) (Byrne & Raphael, 1994; Middleton, Burnett, Raphael, & Martinek, 1996; Prigerson, 2004), which is also called Prolonged Grief Disorder (PGD) (Prigerson et al., 2009). However, the incidence of CG may be even higher (30-50%) when we refer to certain types of death, such as the loss of a child (Keesee, Currier, & Neimeyer, 2008) or the death of a loved one to violent causes (McDevitt-Murphy, Neimeyer, Burke, Williams, & Lawson, 2012). In relation to the symptomatology, and in order to distinguish complicated from normal symptoms, some authors (Horowitz et al., 1993) refer to their intensity and duration. In this sense, high levels of symptoms and a lasting beyond six months post-loss would be a cause of concern (Prigerson, 2004) as well as the total absence of them. However, besides intensity and duration more standards may be used to distinguish pathological from normal grief symptoms, such as statistical, differential symptomatology, and disruption of function criteria (Stroebe et al., 2000). Defining complicated grief is not a simple task. Generally, people struggle deeply and for a prolonged period of time trying to reconstruct a meaningful life without the loved person. Characteristically, CG symptoms include (Shear, Boelen & Neimeyer, 2011): persistent feelings of intense yearning or preoccupation with the deceased, shock, disbelief, and anger about the death; feeling that it is difficult to care for or trust others; and impairing behaviors to try to avoid reminders of the loss or to feel closer to the deceased. In line with this, Prigerson and Jacobs (2001) argue that prolonged grief disorder (PGD) is characterized by intense separation distress, intrusive and emotionally troubling thoughts about the deceased, a sense of meaninglessness, difficulty accepting the loss, and functional impairment.

In view of the different difficulties associated with the complicated grieving process, such as excess risk of mortality and reduction in both physical and psychological health (Stroebe, Schut, & Stroebe, 2007), to identify those bereaved individuals at risk of experiencing important health consequences is an imperative. And further this will enable to carry out an appropriate intervention to prevent negative results wherever possible.

Risk factors have been studied showing that different variables may be related to CG. Nevertheless, this topic needs to be studied with greater depth.

In order to better understand the role of different factors with high health risk consequences during the grieving process, diverse authors have grouped these factors in categories. For example, Sanders (1993) classified them in four categories: biographical/demographic factors, individual factors, type and mode of death, and circumstances following the loss. Likewise, Stroebe and colleagues (Stroebe, Hansson, Stroebe, & Schut, 2001) developed the following categorization: situational factors related to the death, personal factors such as characteristics prior to the death, and interpersonal factors such as the availability of social and emotional support from family and friends.

According to the mentioned authors and in line with Lacasta and Sastre (2000) and Lacasta and Soler (2004) we can summarize the main predictors of CG as associated with the following aspects:

- *Personal*: youth or old age of the bereaved; physical and/or mental previous problems such as depression, anxiety and suicide attempts; previous unresolved grief; inability to cope with stress; very intense reactions of anger, bitterness and guilt; subjective perception of lack of resources to deal with the situation.
- *Relational*: loss of son/daughter, spouse or parent at a young age and/or sibling in adolescence; dependence on the deceased; conflicting or ambivalent relationship with unexpressed hostility.
- *Circumstantial*: deceased youth; sudden and unanticipated loss, accident, homicide, suicide; uncertain and/or multiple deaths; stigmatized death; painful memories during the process.
- *Social or interpersonal*: low socioeconomic status; negative perception or lack of social and family support; responsibility for young children; other stressors such as truncated projects.

Considering this general categorization of possible risk factors for complicated grief as well as the differences found according to the population studied, well known researchers in this field emphasize the outstanding importance of some of the above cited factors. For instance, having a history of psychiatric or medical problems, insecure attachment style, concurrent life stressors, experience multiple important losses, lack of social supports, ambivalent or markedly dependent relationships, sudden and unanticipated death, violent death and the loss of a child (Currier, Holland & Neimeyer, 2006; Johnson, Zhang, Greer, & Prigerson, 2007; Ott, 2003; Rando, 1992; Shear & Mulhare, 2008; Shear & Shair, 2005; Simon et al., 2007; Vanderwerker, Jacobs, Parkes, & Prigerson, 2006). Additionally, other authors include among the main risk factors: cognitions during bereavement (Boelen, Van den Bout, & Van den Hout, 2003a,b), pessimistic temperament and personality correlates (Piper, McCallum, Joyce, Rosie, & Ogrodniczuk, 2001; Robinson & Marwit, 2006). Finally, it is noteworthy that CG or PGD is under consideration for inclusion in the DSM-V as a distinct psychological disorder (Prigerson et al., 2009; Shear et al., 2011), and this fact will improve the management of bereaved individuals undoubtedly. The proposed PGD criteria for the Fifth Edition of the Diagnostic and Statistical Manual of Mental Disorders (Prigerson et al., 2009; Prigerson, Vanderwerker, & Maciejewski, 2008) are:

A. *Event: Bereavement.* The reaction follows the loss of a significant other.
B. *Separation distress.* The bereaved person must experience at least one of the following three symptoms daily or to an intense or disruptive degree: 1) intrusive thoughts related to the deceased; 2) intense pangs of separation distress, or 3) distressingly strong yearnings for that which was lost.
C. *Cognitive, emotional, and behavioral symptoms.* The bereaved person must have five (or more) of the following symptoms experienced daily or to an intense or disruptive degree: 1) confusion about one's role in life or diminished sense of self (i.e., feeling that a part of oneself has died); 2) difficulty accepting the loss; 3) avoidance of reminders of the reality of the loss; 4) inability to trust others since the loss; 5) bitterness or anger related to the loss; 6) difficulty moving on with life (e.g., making new friends, pursuing interests); 7) numbness (absence of emotion) since the loss; 8) feeling that life is unfulfilling, empty, or meaningless since the loss; 9) feeling stunned, dazed or shocked by the loss.
D. *Duration.* Diagnosis should not be made until at least six months have elapsed since the death.
E. *Impairment.* The disturbance causes clinically significant distress or impairment in social, occupational, or other important areas of functioning (e.g., domestic responsibilities).
F. *Relation to other mental disorders.* The disturbance is not better accounted for by major depressive disorder, generalized anxiety disorder, or posttraumatic stress disorder.

Prevention and Treatment

Talking about grief treatment a key question emerges: Is the grief intervention needed by the majority of bereaved individuals? There seems to be general agreement that this is not necessary for a "normal" grieving process (Raphael, Middleton, Martinek, & Misso, 1993; Shear et al., 2011). In line with this, Jordan & Neimeyer (2003) suggest that grief counseling is no "necessary and necessarily helpful for all or most bereaved" (pp. 781) and sometimes could even interfere the grief process.

At this regard, it is of great importance the clinician's knowledge and expertise about bereavement (wide variety of symptoms, boundaries of uncomplicated grief, risk factors for CG, etc.) in order to make the right decision about whether intervene or not (Zisook & Shear, 2009), as well as professionals need to be able to discern what intervention requires each bereaved. That is, the goal could be customize the interventions to the special needs and particularities of each mourner, and above all in those cases with risk factors for complicated grief (Jordan & Neimeyer, 2003).

As noted previously, generally speaking grief is a normal process that does not require specific clinical interventions. However, one of our duties as health professionals will be to facilitate an adaptive course of this process whenever possible.

Particularly in the palliative care field or when we refer to expected deaths, clinicians can act even before the same death. Since the grieving process begins when people are aware of the loss, which may be after receiving the diagnosis and/or prognosis of incurability, bereavement care may start before the death of the loved one and continue beyond.

One of the aims of this attention provided to the bereaved *before the loss* of the loved one is to prevent the onset of a pathological grieving process and to facilitate an adaptive process as far as possible. For this purpose it may be desirable (Arranz, Barbero, Barreto, & Bayés, 2003; Barreto, Molero, & Pérez, 2000; Gil-Juliá, Bellver & Ballester, 2008; Lacasta & Sastre, 2000): to promote in the relatives the expression of feelings, the conservation of other roles different to the caregiver, an active role in the care and symptom control, the breakdown of a maladaptive denial when this compromise the patient care, the rupture of the conspiracy of silence if there is no an adaptive denial by the patient, and the end of an important lack of emotional communication. Moreover, to increase the sense of usefulness,to help in the distribution of tasks among family members so that everyone could feel well involved in the patient's care, to explore fears, to prepare a practical organization just in case the relative could be alone at the time of death, to allow the patient's chance of choosing with whom to die (when possible), to find solution to the pending practical and/or emotional issues. In addition to normalize those feelings and thoughts that may lead to the bereaved to subsequent guilt (for example, come to desire that the patient will die or experience relief when they die, are normal feelings when death cannot be avoided and the care process has gone on for months), and to facilitate those rituals that help the family to say goodbye to the beloved.

To facilitate the understanding of the content just quoted, all these aspects could be summarized in five categories, as follows: 1) to identify the relatives' needs, problems, concerns and fears in order to suppress or relieve them, 2) to assess and enhance the resources of the family in order to better manage their emotions, thoughts and behaviors, while attempting to reduce the feeling of impotence and to increase the control over the situation, 3) to assess risk factors and to prevent possible complications whilst offering alternatives, 4) to provide the family with the proper information and 5) to help relatives in the acceptance of the patient's near future, that is, his death.

At this point, *after the death* of the loved one, clinicians will continue their work in terms of prevention of a pathological process and promoting the adaptation to the changing reality. It is worth bearing in mind that the attention provided hereafter will focused on those bereaved at risk for complicated grief as well as those bereaved who request attention because of their lack of resources' self-perception to cope with the current situation properly. Some of the goals to be achieved would be (Barreto & Soler, 2007; Gil-Juliá et al., 2008; Neimeyer, Baldwin, & Gillies, 2006; Parkes & Weiss, 1983): to facilitate all those aspects that could lead to acknowledge the reality of the loss, to provide information about the grieving process, to tackle the circumstances of the death (clarifying confusing events), to talk about the history of the lost relationship (reviewing both positive and negative issues), to fulfill unfinished business, to strengthen the existing adaptive elements, to promote an appropriate expression of thoughts, feelings and emotions (sadness, anxiety, anger, rage and guilt), to promote the gradual adaptation to the new situation, to identify effective support or its absence among family and friends, to increase social support, to help the bereaved both, to rebuild a new relationship with the deceased person in a compatible way with the current reality and to search for meaning in the wake of the loss.

Likewise, it is of key importance to identify those individuals with complicated grief in order to provide them a specialized intervention, which may be necessary to help the mourner move forward.

There are a wide range of techniques on which clinicians can draw in their work with bereaved people. Some of the most widely used techniques in this context are listed below (Gil-Juliá et al., 2008; Lacasta & de Luis, 2002; Lacasta & Sastre, 2000; Worden, 1997):

- Using letters, diaries, photos, poetry and visualization to express emotions, thoughts, memories, reconciliation, to say goodbye and to give personal meaning to the experience of loss.
- Using different resources such as photos, videos and paintings to stimulate memories and emotions.
- "Role playing" helps people to play different roles related to fearful or uncomfortable situations, allowing the bereaved to learn skills and coping strategies.
- Visualization and imagination foster the integration of the loss. They promote the expression of feelings and thoughts and may be used as a means of reconciliation and farewell. The empty chair technique has been also proved very useful. The key of its success is no the imagination but to be in the present and to speak to the deceased instead of talking about him.
- Cognitive restructuring to change negative unhelpful cognitions. The goal is identifying, discussing and changing those negative thoughts, which are interfering with an adaptive grieving process.
- Problem solving approach facilitates appropriate decision making.
- Thought stopping, when they cause anxiety and are not productive.
- Contingency management: reinforcement of adaptive behaviors and extinction of maladaptive ones.
- Relaxation techniques for anxiety and insomnia situations.
- Planning rewarding activities and management of social skills.

All this without forgetting that one of the most important aspects related to the use of the different techniques is to choose the right time and to take into account the particularities of each individual.

For an extensive understanding of creative techniques for counseling the bereaved, the reader may consult a recent book entitled "Techniques of Grief therapy" edited by Neimeyer (2012).

Grief is a natural and universal process in response to the loss characterized by peaks and valleys. It is worth underscoring the importance of well knowing this process to avoid significant mistakes such as over or under-diagnosis, either pathologizing a normal and adaptive condition or failing to treat a disorder. And in line with Jordan and Neimeyer (2003) we also believe that a key element in this process is the relationship between the bereaved and the clinician, who should be always in tune with the first providing a healing experience with total respect, understanding and compassionate empathy.

REFERENCES

Arranz, P., Barbero, J. J., Barreto, P. & Bayés, R. (2003). *Intervención emocional en Cuidados Paliativos.Protocolos deintervención*. Barcelona: Ariel.

Barreto, M. P., Molero, M. & Pérez, M. A. (2000). Evaluación e intervención psicológica en familias de enfermos oncológicos. In F. Gil (Ed.), *Manual de psicooncología* (137-171). Madrid: Nova Sidonia Oncología.

Barreto, P. & Soler, M. C. (2007). *Muerte y duelo*. Madrid: Síntesis.

Boelen, P. A. & Prigerson, H. G. (2007). The influence of symptoms of prolonged grief disorder, depression, and anxiety on quality of life bereaved adults: A prospective study. *European Arch. Psychiatry Clinical Neuroscience*, *257*, 444-452.

Boelen, P. A., Van den Bout, J. & Van den Hout, M. A. (2003a). The role of negative interpretations of grief reactions in emotional problems after bereavement. *Journal of Behavior Therapy and Experimental Psychiatry*, *34*, 225-238.

Boelen, P. A., Van den Bout, J. & Van den Hout, M. A. (2003b). The role of cognitive variables in psychological functioning after the death of a first degree relative. *Behaviour Research and Therapy*, *41*, 1123-1136.

Bonanno, G. A. & Boerner, K. (2007). The stage theory of grief. *JAMA*, *297*, 2693.

Bonanno, G. A., Wortman, C. B. & Nesse, R. M. (2004). Prospective patterns of resilience and maladjustment during widowhood. *Psychology and Aging*, *19*, 260-271.

Bowlby, J. (1961). Processes of mourning. *International Journal of Psychoanalysis*, *42*, 317-339.

Bowlby, J. (1980). Loss: Sadness and depression. New York: Basic Books.

Byrne, G. J. & Raphael, B. (1994). A longitudinal study of bereavement phenomena in recently widowed elderly men. *Psychological Medicine*, *24*, 411-421.

Currier, J. M., Holland, J. M. & Neimeyer, R. A. (2006). Sense-Making, Grief, and the Experience of Violent Loss: Toward a Mediational Model. *Death Studies*, *30*, 403-428.

Engel, G. (1964). Grief and grieving. *American Journal of Nursing*, *64*, 93-98.

Gil-Juliá, B., Bellver, A. & Ballester, R. (2008). Duelo: evaluación, diagnóstico y tratamiento. *Psicooncología*, *5*, 103-116.

Glick, I. O., Weiss, R. S. & Parkes, C. M. (1974). The first year of bereavement. New York: Wiley.

Holland, J. M. & Neimeyer, R. A. (2010). An Examination of Stage Theory of Grief among Individuals Bereaved by Natural and Violent Causes: A Meaning-Oriented Contribution. *OMEGA, Journal of Death and Dying*, *61*, 103-120.

Horowitz, M. J., Stinson, C. H., Fridhandler, B., Milbrath, C., Redington, D., & Ewert, M. (1993). Pathological grief: An intensive case study. *Psychiatry, Interpersonal and Biological Processes*, *56*, 356-374.

Jacobs, S., Hansen, F., Kasl, S., Ostfeld, A., Berkman, L. & Kim, K. (1990). Anxiety disorders during acute bereavement: Risk and risk factors. *Journal of Clinical Psychiatry*, *51*, 269-274.

Johnson, J. G., Zhang, B., Greer, J. A. & Prigerson, H. G. (2007). Parental control, partner dependency, and complicated grief among widowed adults in the community. *The Journal of Nervous and Mental Disease*, *195*, 26-30.

Jordan, J. R. & Neimeyer, R. A. (2003). Does grief counseling work? *Death Studies*, *27*, 765-786.

Keesee, N. J., Currier, J. M. & Neimeyer, R. A. (2008). Predictors of Grief Following the Death of One's Child: The Contribution of Finding Meaning. *Journal of Clinical Psychology*, *64*, 1145-1163.

Kübler-Ross, E. (1969). *On Death and Dying*. New York, NY: Macmillan.

Lacasta, M. A., & de Luis, V. (2002). Evaluación de los resultados a largo plazo de un programa de atención al duelo. *Revista de la Sociedad Española del Dolor*, *9*, 502-509.

Lacasta, M. A., & Sastre, P. (2000). El manejo del duelo. In M. Die, & E. López (Eds.), *Aspectos psicológicos en cuidados paliativos. La comunicación con el enfermo y la familia* (491-506). Madrid: Ades Ediciones.

Lacasta, M. A. & Soler, M. C. (2004). El duelo: prevención y tratamiento del duelo patológico. Cuidados después de la muerte. In C. Camps, J. Carrulla, A. Casas, M. González Barón, J. Sanz, & V. Valentín (Eds.), *Manual SEOM de Cuidados Continuos* (713-730). Madrid: Dispublic, SL.

Latiegi, A. (1999). Prevención y tratamiento del duelo patológico. In W. Astudillo, C. Arrieta, C. Mendinueta, & I. Vega de Seoane (Eds.), *La familia en la terminalidad* (295-313). San Sebastián: Sociedad Vasca de Cuidados Paliativos.

Lindemann, E. (1944). Symptomatology and management of acute grief. *American Journal of Psychiatry*, *101*, 141-148.

Maciejewski, P. K., Zhang, B., Block, S. D. & Prigerson, H. G. (2007). An Empirical Examination of the Stage Theory of Grief. *JAMA*, *297*, 716-723.

McDevitt-Murphy, M. E., Neimeyer, R. A., Burke, L. A., Williams, J. L. & Lawson, K. (2012). The toll of traumatic loss in African Americans bereaved by homicide. *Psychological Trauma: Theory, Research, Practice, and Policy*, *4*, 303-311. DOI: 10.1037/a0024911.

Middleton, W., Burnett, P., Raphael, B. & Martinek, N. (1996). The bereavement response: A cluster analysis. *The British Journal of Psychiatry*, *169*, 167-171.

Neimeyer, R. A. (2008). Prolonged grief disorder. In C. Bryant and D. Peck (Eds.), *Encyclopedia of death and the human experience*. Thousand Oaks, CA: Sage.

Neimeyer, R. A. (2012). *Techniques of Grief Therapy*. New York: Routledge.

Neimeyer, R. A., Baldwin, S. A. & Gillies, J. (2006). Continuing bonds and reconstructing meaning: mitigating complications in bereavement. *Death Studies*, *30*, 715-738.

Ott, C. H. (2003). The impact of complicated grief on mental and physical health at various points in the bereavement process. *Death Studies*, *27*, 249-272.

Parkes, C. (1972). Bereavement: Studies in Grief in Adult Life. London, England: Tavistock.

Parkes, C. M. & Weiss, R. S. (1983). *Recovery from bereavement*. New York: Basic Books.

Piper, W. E., McCallum, M., Joyce, A. S., Rosie, J. S. & Ogrodniczuk, J. S. (2001). Patient personality and time-limited group psychotherapy for complicated grief. *International Journal of Group Psychotherapy*, *51*, 525-552.

Prigerson, H. G. (2004). Complicated grief. *Bereavement Care*, *23*, 38-40.

Prigerson, H., Frank, E., Kasl, S., Reynolds, C., III, Anderson, B. & Zubenko, G. et al. (1995). Complicated grief and bereavement-related depression as distinct disorders: Preliminary empirical validation in elderly bereaved spouses. *American Journal of Psychiatry*, *152*, 22-30.

Prigerson, H. G., Horowitz, M. J., Jacobs, S. C., Parkes, C. M., Aslan, M. & Goodkin, K. et al. (2009). Prolonged grief disorder: Psychometric validation of criteria proposed for DSM-V and ICD-11. *PloS Medicine*, *6*, e1000121. doi:10. 1371/journal. pmed. 1000121.

Prigerson, H. G. & Jacobs, S. C. (2001). Diagnostic criteria for traumatic grief: A rationale, consensus criteria, and a preliminary empirical test. In M. S.

Stroebe, R. O. Hansson, W. Stroebe, & H. Schut (Eds.), *Handbook of bereavement research: Consequences, coping, and care* (613-645). Washington, DC: American Psychological Association.

Prigerson, H. G. & Maciejewski, P. K. (2008). Grief and acceptance as opposite sides of the same coin: setting a research agenda to study peaceful acceptance of loss. *The British Journal of Psychiatry*, *193*, 435-437. doi: 10. 1192/bjp. bp. 108. 053157.

Prigerson, H. G., Vanderwerker, L. C. & Maciejewski, P. K. (2008). A case for inclusion of prolonged grief disorder in DSM–V. In M. Stroebe, R. Hansson, H. Schut, & W. Stroebe (Eds.), *Handbook of bereavement research and practice: Advances in theory and intervention* (165-186). Washington, DC: American Psychological Association.

Rando, T. A. (1984). Grief, dying and death. *Clinical interventions for caregivers*. Champaign (IL): Champaign Press.

Rando, T. (1992). The increasing prevalence of complicated mourning: the onslaught is just beginning. *Omega-Journal of death and dying*, *26*, 43-59.

Raphael, B., Middleton, W., Martinek, N. & Misso, V. (1993). Counseling and therapy of the bereaved. In M. Stroebe, W. Stroebe & R. O. Hansson (Eds.), *Handbook of bereavement: Theory, research and intervention* (427-453). Cambridge, England: Cambridge University Press.

Robinson, T. & Marwit, S. J. (2006). An investigation of the relationship of personality, coping, and grief intensity among bereaved mothers. *Death Studies*, *30*, 677-696.

Sanders, C. M. (1993). Risk factors in bereavement outcome. In M. Stroebe, W. Stroebe & R. O. Hansson (Eds.), *Handbook of bereavement: Theory, research and intervention* (255-267). Cambridge, England: Cambridge University Press.

Schut, H. A. W., de Keijser, J., van den Bout, J. & Dijkhuis, J. H. (1991). Post-traumatic stress symptoms in the first year of conjugal bereavement. *Anxiety Research*, *4*, 225-234.

Shear, M. K., Boelen, P. A. & Neimeyer, R. A. (2011). Treating Complicated Grief. Converging Approaches. In R. A. Neimeyer, D. L. Harris, H. R. Winokuer & G. F. Thornton (Eds.), *Grief and Bereavement in Contemporary Society. Bridging research and practice* (139-162). New York: Routledge.

Shear, M. K. & Mulhare, E. (2008). Complicated grief. *Psychiatric Annals*, *38*, 662-670.

Shear, K. & Shair, H. (2005). Attachment, loss, and complicated grief. *Developmental Psychobiology*, *47*, 253-267.

Shear, M. K., Simon, N., Wall, M. Zisook, S., Neimeyer, R. & Duan, N. et al. (2011). Complicated grief and related bereavement issues for DSM-5. *Depression and Anxiety*, *28*, 103-117.

Silver, R. C. & Wortman, C. B. (2007). The stage theory of grief. *JAMA*, *297*, 2692.

Simon, N. M., Shear, K. M., Thompson, E. H., Zalta, A. K., Perlman, C., Reynolds, C. F. Frank, E., Melhem, N. M. & Silowash, R. (2007). The prevalence and correlates of psychiatric comorbidity in individuals with complicated grief. *Comprehensive Psychiatry*, *48*, 395-399.

Shuchter, S. R. & Zisook, S. (1993). The course of normal grief. In M. S. Stroebe, W. Stroebe, & R. O. Hansson (Eds.), *Handbook of bereavement: Theory, research and intervention* (23-43). Cambridge, England: Cambridge University Press.

Stroebe, M., Hansson, R. O., Stroebe, W. & Schut, H. (2001). *Handbook of bereavement research.* Washington, DC: American Psychological Association.

Stroebe, M., Schut, H. & Stroebe, W. (2007). Health outcomes of bereavement. *Lancet*, *370*, 1960-1973.

Stroebe, M., van Son, M., Stroebe, W., Kleber, R., Schut, H. & van den Bout, J. (2000). On the classification and diagnosis of pathological grief. *Clinical Psychology Review*, *20*, 57-75.

Vanderwerker, L. C., Jacobs, S. C., Parkes, C. M. & Prigerson, H. G. (2006). An exploration of associations between separation anxiety in childhood and complicated grief in later life. *The Journal of Nervous and Mental Disease*, *194*, 121-123.

Worden, J. W. (1997). *El tratamiento del duelo.* Barcelona: Paidós.

Worden, W. (1982). *Grief counseling and grief therapy.* New York: Springer.

Worden, J. W. & Winokuer, H. R. (2011). A Task-Based Approach for Counseling the Bereaved. In R. A. Neimeyer, D. L. Harris, H. R. Winokuer & G. F. Thornton (Eds.), *Grief and Bereavement in Contemporary Society. Bridging research and practice* (57-67). New York: Routledge.

Zisook, S. & Shear, K. (2009). Grief and bereavement: what psychiatrists need to know. *World Psychiatry*, *8*, 67-74.

Zisook, S., Shuchter, S. R., Sledge, P. A., Paulus, M. & Judd, L. W. (1994). The spectrum of depressive phenomena after spousal bereavement. *Journal of Clinical Psychiatry*, *55*, 29-36.

In: End-of-Life Care
Editors: Maria Rossi and Luiz Ortiz
ISBN: 978-1-62808-555-6

Chapter 5

CARE FOR DYING PATIENTS: MULTIDIMENSIONAL ASPECTS OF NURSING CARE

Małgorzata Pasek[1,2,*], Grażyna Osuch-Pęcak[1] and Maciej Krajewski[3]

[1]Centre of Oncology – Maria Sklodowska-Curie Memorial Institute, Cracow Division, Poland

[2]Institute of Health Care, Higher Vocational School in Tarnów, Poland

[3]The Greater Poland Cancer Centre in Poznan, Poland

ABSTRACT

Human death is a mystery. Although scientists have identified the criteria, states, and signs of biological death, undoubtedly the issues of dying and death have a wider meaning.

In this paper we would like to emphasize the multidimensional character of the process of dying and nursing care offered during this period. This type of care is tightly associated with various ethical problems and dilemmas. This results from subjectively assessed health-related quality of life, among others. The dilemmas pertain to patient's expectations and decisions made by his/her loved ones or the members of therapeutic team. Starting another regimen of anticancer treatment and reducing the dose of pain medications in order to avoid addiction, the

* Corresponding author: Email: malgorzata_pasek@wp.pl.

patient meets the expectations of his/her loved ones; frequently these expectations represent unmitigated fight for life. Is such attitude always beneficial for the patient? The lack of universal solutions is reflected by various controversies pertaining both to the crucial decisions and to the selection of the methods and way of care.

Nursing care is related to all dimensions of human being: biological, psychological, social, spiritual, and cultural ones. The care should be offered both to the dying patient and to his/her loved ones.

Esteem, friendliness, empathy, openness, as well as the ability and accuracy of responding to somatic suffering seem to be both the source of support and the sign of care for a patient and his/her family.

Professional career of a nurse comprises various stages associated with realizing her abilities with regards to life, dying, and death. The professionalism of a nurse can be manifested by her creative presence, care, assistance, and consolation; however, it is not always possible to get rid of the feeling of helplessness, lack of acceptance to passing away, and other strong emotions in view of patient's death.

During this study we talked to terminally-ill patients of a hospice. This research confirmed that every human being dies differently. We have been surprised by various attitudes to death, as well as by different expectations toward accompanying persons. Not only each dying person is different as an individual, also his/her mood and mental status change rapidly and sometimes unexpectedly. Also this finding emphasizes the importance and difficulties associated with care for terminally-ill patients.

The above mentioned observations suggest that despite nurses' experience in accompanying dying individuals, one should not create any universal model of care for this group of patients.

In the philosophical context, everything which is experienced by human being during his/her life is unique and happens only once. Even if we perceive our life as monotonous and following a reproducible scheme, none of situations, events, or relationships we experience never prove to be the same.

Also death, including the clinical cases, happens only once. It cannot be repeated, as well as we are unable to prepare better for this event, deepen our relationships with our close relatives, or accept more of their support. Similarly, we cannot make the general rehearsal of our death, or master its course.

There is not one optimal standard of dying and death. This statement is true both in case of dying individuals and their families, as well as in the case of individuals who offer them professional care.

However, despite the irreproducibility of death, one can prepare for participation and assistance in care for dying individuals and their families.

This preparation includes improving general and professional knowledge, especially in such disciplines as philosophy, psychology, oncology and palliative care, as well as oncological and palliative nursing. Mastering skills and attitudes can be supported by participation in workshops and courses, as well as by studying relevant literature (e.g. publications presenting experiences of nurses and other professionals offering care for dying individuals, or diaries of patients and their families).

In Poland, the care for dying patients is affected with many stigmas. They mostly pertain to the tabuization of death and dying. Although most individuals declare that death is the only certain thing in our life, it is considered as rather unreal and distant phenomenon in everyday practice. Moreover, during their high school education, future doctors are imbued that most deaths correspond to failure or lost fight with a disease.

According to WHO, improving the life quality of terminally ill patients and their families constitutes the principal objective of palliative care. The quality of life is defined as a self-perceived situation in a given period of time[1]. In the case of dying individuals, this can pertain to four areas: 1/ motor skill, manifested as ability to self-care, 2/ somatic status, described in terms of experienced symptoms and ability to control them, 3/ mental status, describing the extent of acceptance and adaptation to current conditions, and the presence of positive and negative emotions, and 4/ social status, reflecting the type and quality of interpersonal relationships. Studies of the quality of life of terminally ill patients may raise many controversies, including the ethical dilemmas. The two ideas are confronted. One would like to offer the patient and his/her family the optimal and satisfying care. However, one should consider the suffering of terminally ill patient, the fragility of his/her existence, helplessness, and the fact that not infrequently he or she concentrates on internal emotions and drifts away from the world of living people.

Consequently, these two components should be combined, and the methods of care which manifest respect for the dignity of dying individual and his/her family should be sought.

The aim of this paper is to present the selected aspects of nursing care for dying individuals. We present the opinions of patients (R), as well as the attitudes of the members of their families and caregivers (O) in order to provide more comprehensive insight in the problem in question. The study was

[1] de Walden – Gałuszko K., Majkowicz M., Model oceny jakości opieki paliatywnej realizowanej w warunkach stacjonarnych. Zakład Medycyny Paliatywnej AMG, Gdańsk 2001

conducted in a hospice for adults in Cracow, and was based on a diagnostic survey. We used the technique of open interview. The participation in the study was anonymous. Prior to the interview, the clinical status of patients was determined, and an informed consent to participate in the study was sought.

Amongst various attitudes towards care for dying individuals, there are two which can raise particular concerns. The first of them is characterized by the lack of empathy, and ignorance to problems; it frequently results from the fear of death itself. This manifests as persuading the suffering individual that his/her pain is unavoidable and nothing can be done to alleviate it. The second attitude is associated with conviction that the care offered to patient and his/her family is optimal or even ideal. *Our patients do not suffer, do not experience pain; both they and their families are offered holistic care.* Such statement, being nothing more than wishful thinking, results in an ignorance to the real needs and problems of dying individual and his/her family. Too optimistic self-assessment of one's abilities and skills, and the lack of current diagnosis, analysis and conclusions related to care for patient and his/her family can be reflected by inadvertent routine. As a result, the subject of care is not considered the highest and most important value, but this is rather the care itself which is affirmed.

Moreover, the problems associated with care offered to dying individual and his/her family are also related to the awareness of approaching death. In their concept, B.G. Glaser and A.L. Strauss[2] defined four types of awareness which modulate the extent and quality of interaction between the dying individual and the others. These include: 1/ closed awareness, when the patient is kept ignorant of his/her terminal status, while his/her family and the others are well aware of it, 2/ suspicion awareness, when the terminally ill patient suspects his/her situation and tries to obtain any information, 3/ mutual pretence, when both the patient and his/her close relatives are well aware of the truth but pretend being ignorant of it, and 4/ open awareness, when both parties are aware of the situation and discuss it openly.

Probably, the situation in which the true status of the patient is revealed, along with the short-term prognosis, and relationships with his/her closest relatives, constitutes the optimal model. However, our interviews with individuals taking care for terminally ill patients suggest that they do not always want to talk about death:

[2] Ostrowska A., Śmierć w doświadczeniu jednostki i społeczeństwa, wyd IFiS PAN, Warzawa 2005, , s. 141.

> O: No, rather not. Rarely, some of them realize this fact. Others try to ignore it. Some faithful patients stop praying and condemn the God for everything, or irritate themselves "why me?" My reply is "why not?", everyone can die tomorrow, a day after tomorrow, or in a week; we have to accept it. There is something in human nature that we get rid of bad thoughts, and cheat ourselves.
>
> O: Very rarely. Most of them do not realize their status or do not want to realize it. They plan to recover and leave this place. I remember being astonished with this observation. After completing my hospice volunteer course, I expected being asked such questions, but it is just opposite.
>
> O: Rarely. Some patients have such need and ask many questions, but this is minority. Most of them are afraid of discussing the problem.
>
> O: No, I did not observe it. Maybe rather with a priest or psychologist; with us rarely. The only thing they say is "I am dying"; their realize it, and perhaps expect us to negate it and say that it is still not the time; however, we do not do so, we do not give them a false hope. If the patient asks difficult questions we seek for psychologist, but some of the patients choose nurse as a partner in discussion.

Another group of our responders emphasized the role of the balance of life; if it is positive, it is easier for the patient to discuss about his/her death, and to accept it. It can be concluded that individuals who accepted their death, can discuss it without emotions:

> O: Some of them would like but they are afraid of. The fear of death has many components. Each of us possess the instinct of self-protection. We are afraid of unknown. Individuals who pass away with a negative balance of their life, are usually afraid of death. If the balance is positive, the death is usually calm. Older individuals show more acceptance to death, they believe that they had lived long enough and it is the time to pass away; obviously, not everybody. In contrast, younger patients cannot accept their death. It is not natural.

Anxiety, fear, and uncertainty represent emotions and states which are frequently experienced by an individual facing the necessity of his/her death. Death is the end of life but also represents its vastness, as a transition, mystery, and unknown. Although people are afraid of death, sometimes their worry that death has forgotten about them (especially if they are tired, exhausted with life, senility, or chronic conditions). There are people who are ready for death, wait for it, or even want it to come.

Studies of the specialists in noo-logotherapy[3] revealed that the individuals who are creatively involved in their life represent creative values. The feeling of good and meaningful life let them to experience suffering creatively. Obviously, does not mean that physical pain or suffering are lower; nevertheless, there are ascribed different meaning. However, despair and hopelessness constitute predominant emotions in individuals whose life is characterized by negative values.

During our discussions with the patients of Cracow hospice we observed that some of them limited to answering particular questions; they did not self-analyze their experiences related to death, and avoided them. They more eagerly discussed others' deaths rather that their own death, as it was not related to themselves.

> R: When I was admitted, a patient died in this room. I thought that I have brought him death. None have died in my presence before. Subsequently, other two patients died. They died calmly. One had fallen unwell and then fell asleep. Another one was lying in his bed, and died at noon; he had lung cancer but was kept ignorant of it. His family members did not want him to know.

Another group of patients talked about death with anxiety and fear of unknown. Nevertheless, also this group comprised individuals in whom hope mixed with despair:

> R: Yes. I took part in the funeral of my sister and brother; I did not attend my husband's funeral as we were divorced. This rather did not influence my way of thinking. I simply do not think about death, consider it distant; what will happen, will happen. I am well aware of the disease progression. But sometimes I forget that I am terminally ill, I have a lot of hope. But sometimes again the blues comes /she is crying/ and I am unable to fight it. I am mentally strong but my disease results from my stressful life.
>
> R: Yes, I have experienced it. But it is different if somebody dies suddenly rather than being chronically ill, and get used to dying. I am afraid of death as it is unknown route.

It often happens, as reported by M. Adamczak[4], that the terminally ill patient is aware of approaching end of life, and experiences despair; however,

[3] Suchocka L., Psychologia bólu, Wydawnictwo Difin, Warszawa 2008.

[4] Adamczak M., Psychospołeczne problemy chorego terminalnie i jego rodziny, [w:] Drążkiewicz J., W stronę człowieka umierającego, UW Warszawa 1989, s. 55.

he or she still hopes that the faith will change, and represents wishful thinking with regards to his/her status. Therefore, such person lives in two domains: real one – frightening, and irrational one – alleviating.

The anxiety experienced by the dying individual and his/her close relatives is not an usual fear of something unknown . In the case of approaching death, it is rather the feeling of helplessness in the confrontation with the inevitable loss of the most precious value. It is a paralyzing anxiety against the destruction of human body and mind. According to psycho-oncologists, the studies of emotions experienced by terminally ill individuals, although initially only in theory (until experienced personally, e.g. dying and death of a close relative, which we at least partly co-experience), seem necessary as they provide more mindful assistance and contact with our patients. While the ignorance of somatic and mental processes associated with dying can enhance the fears of caregiver, or even make him/her reluctant to entering the room of the terminally ill person, the lack of information and apparent avoidance of contact with dying patient enhance the feeling of loneliness anxiety of the latter.

Other responses suggest that death is frequently equaled to suffering, and this is the suffering which raises most of the fears. While death is an abstract term, the suffering is tangible and experienced:

> R: I thought about death earlier. Not that I will die, but rather in general; therefore it is nothing new to me. Nevertheless, I do not know what will happen when I will face it; I do not know how I will behave. It is the worst if you lie in bed and nothing help; it is terrible. I am faithful, but my faith is rational; thus, I do not believe that one has to suffer. But I you suffer, you have not choice – you have to bear it.
>
> R: My husband knew that it will come but tried to ignore it. He was afraid of death and did not talk about it; therefore, also I have not discussed the problem although I realized that I got used to it. He was afraid of what will happen; he asked his doctor about it. He wanted to know if he suffer; he was afraid of suffering.

Additionally, death and dying have biological dimension. The presence of clinical symptoms and discomfort can exert significant impact on the quality of passing away.

The diagnosis of dying is based on the presence of such symptoms as excessive respiratory discharge, pain, restlessness/fear, dyspnea, nausea, and vomiting. Moreover, patients with advanced cancers may show progressive weakness, decreased activity (staying in bed, lack of independence in most self-care activities), reduced ingestion of foods and fluids, sleepiness, impaired consciousness, lack of interest, and swallowing disorders including problems in taking oral medications[5]. Correct identification of so-called point with no return determines the discontinuation of extensive treatment, and protects the patient against additional unnecessary suffering.

The period of agony is associated with the aggravation of dying signs. These signs include problems with breathing, sharpening of facial line, strong pain, nervousness and restlessness, loss of consciousness, dyspnea, and xerostomy.

The principal objectives of treatment implemented during dying and agony include the attenuation of symptoms; however, one should screen the balance between the control of symptoms and the side effects of applied symptomatic treatment. The type of planned treatment can / should be discussed with the patient. Some patients prefer remaining conscious despite the presence of unbearable symptoms, while the others decide upon immediate sedative treatment. However, it should be remembered that the patient can always change his/her opinion.

Problem of pain occupies central position in patients' minds. Even if the pain was controlled, it is sometimes so unforgettable that one cannot stop thinking about it. According to a definition, the somatic pain is an unpleasant sensation resulting from the stimuli causing the injury of tissues or associated with the risk of their injury. Although usually the pain is treated pharmacologically, also providing proper environment, i.e. silence and the feeling of safety, is vitally important[6].

> R: You know, they say that they can control the pain, but is it really true? I am afraid of it but I know that they will do their best to help me. I was still not affected by pain today. I also suffer from diabetes but it is not really a problem.
>
> R: Obviously, I experience pain; I am given analgesics, but still feel some pain. I am worrying that this pain will exacerbate and would like it to be reduced. The pain is most important problem; I do not experience any other symptoms. I lie in bed as I am unable to walk. Sometimes I move on a wheelchair; it depends on the availability of medical personnel and my status. But this is not the worst; this is the pain I am still most afraid of.

---

[5] Kinghorn S., Gaines S., Opieka Paliatywna, Wydawnictwo Elsevier Urban&Partner, Wrocław 2012

[6] Winkler B., Ból nowotworowy jako zjawisko somatopsychiczne, [w:] Problemy medycyny paliatywnej, Praca zbiorowa, Lublin 1996, s. 69–73.

Imposing our opinion on the patient, e.g. saying "you should not use too many analgesics as you can become addicted", "you cannot give up", "you should undertake another attempt of treatment or other life-saving procedures", seems unacceptable. However, this may happen if the members of family do not accept their close relative to pass away. The motivation to life and survival by all means is not necessarily consistent with real abilities and needs of the patient.

The so-called following patient's awareness and will is one prerequisite of advisable and ethical care for dying individuals. However, this requires setting a relationship with the patient; this gives us an opportunity to reveal what he/she truly knows about his/her status and what are his/her imaginations in this matter, to which extent he/she would like to be informed, and what are his/her worries and expectations (e.g. with regards to medical professionals). Optimal, proper care for dying patient seems impossible without the effort to know him/her truly[7] (providing his/her allowance to do so), and facing his/her difficult emotions. These objectives cannot be met if contact with the patient is limited to the administration of sedatives and analgesics.

Satisfying the need for safety is an important component of care. It is also associated with the feeling of hope. A term "total pain" exists in palliative care; this refers to the pain which is experienced not only in its somatic aspect, but has also psychological, social and spiritual background. It is diagnosed whenever the lost sense of life and the lack of hope predominate amongst patient's emotions.

The awareness of being a problem for the others constitutes a factor negatively affects the feeling of social safety. It is also one reason listed amongst the potential causes of euthanasia. During our interviews we tried to reveal if terminally ill patients perceive themselves as a problem for the others and suffer due to this awareness. This question was addressed solely to the members of patients' families and their caregivers.

Some of the responders did not realize the problem in question:

> O: No, he never perceived himself as a problem, and still believed that he will survive. Indeed, he was aware that he will die one day, but still fought and believed that it was not the time.
>
> O: No, rather not. They are happy that somebody assists them. They do not perceive themselves as a problem for the others; this rather is not an issue in the case of dying patients.

---

[7] Kępiński A., Poznanie chorego, Wydawnictwo Literackie, Kraków 2002.

The other group of responders emphasized the occurrence of such problems, and mentioned various reasons behind this situation. Some of the responders pointed to the fact that many patients live alone. The others suggested that the disease-related dependence from the others represents the negation of earlier life in the case of previously independent individuals. Their role in the family changes and not infrequently it is easier for them to accept help from the strangers than from their closest relatives:

> O: Yes, I sometimes face it. They say that it is unnecessary as it will not help. This attitude is frequently presented by lonely people who lost the sense of their life and believe that nobody needs them.
>
> O: It happens, but rarely. These are patients who wanted to be unproblematic throughout their entire life. These are difficult patients. They will never disclose their suffering, we have to force them to admit that they suffer. We frequently hear: "Nurse, you do not have to work so hard; I am old". But we persuade them to disclose their problems since we want to help them.
>
> O: It happens, but depends on the patient's status. We do not experience it with patients who are independent. However, those whom we have to change diapers, lift or feed them frequently say: "How much work you have with me!", "Why I am here?", "I will die nevertheless".
>
> O: Yes, they say so but in various context. Sometimes they are ashamed of being a problem to their close relatives; they do not accept help from their families, and this is one reason behind their referral to the Hospice. Patients are afraid of losing their power, strength, feeling of control, but also their intimacy. This is the cause of the problem in question rather than the fact that they are rebuffed by anyone. It is easier to accept help for a stranger than from a family member. We try to convince them that they can be helpful for us in many aspects, seek for any activities for them, define them small objectives in order to activate them. This is searching for alternative spheres of self-realization. They have to perceive themselves necessary. Sometimes the problem enhances if the patient does his/her best to stop being a problem for his/her family.

Another responder highlighted another dimension of hope, as she emphasized the switch of objectives. This latter term corresponds to the ability of enjoying with small pleasures; as a result, the loss of hope for recovery does not necessarily correspond to a drama:

> O: We do not strain ourselves to talk about hope; instead, we give the real hope. We do not lie to our patients, but want them to think realistically. We give them a chance to prepare for dying. They should switch their objectives; instead of thinking about going on vacation they

should enjoy with meeting their families, agreement with their relatives. They should accept their disease; this is really important. This is our success: they accepted their status despite the lack of chances for recovery. The hope of recovery is not always recommended, in contrast to hope in general, e.g. one should hope that he/she will not suffer or that he/she will not be alone.

The conceptual model of hope in palliative care includes three concepts: comfort, attachment, and value. Comfort pertains to concentration on activities which can raise and maintain hope. This refers mostly to the efficient coping somatic symptoms as they can enhance the despair of patients and their families. The concepts of attachment emphasizes the importance of contact with the others, particularly in cases in which an advanced disease with unfavorable prognosis is associated with uncertainty and fear. Many individuals are afraid of being abandoned, isolated, and lacking support. Finally, the concept of value highlights the importance of patient and his/her family as individual and unique entities. Proper communication and the feeling of the sense of life and its objectives modulate the quality of life. Therefore, these three co-existing components act synergistically[8].

The care for dying individuals and their families cannot be limited to the act of spontaneous activity of medical personnel and other individuals of good will. Many countries developed the policy of integrated care for people who die. For example, an order to provide high-quality care for all dying patients and their families was formulated by the British government in 2000. Among others, this pertained to the implementation of LCP policy, i.e. the Liverpool Care Pathway for the dying patients. Multidisciplinary task forces were organized, including nurses, specialists for palliative and pastoral care, pharmacists, social care workers, and the coordinators of integrated care pathways (ICPs)[9].

The LCP comprises three stages. The initial assessment of patient's needs and the needs of his/her family and the implementation of proper care are aimed at providing comfort for the terminally ill individual, as well as at defining the need and extent of further medical and nursing activities. Further stages include the promotion of proper communication, providing information to patients, their families, and other individuals who are involved in care, and

[8] Kinghorn S., Gaines S., Opieka Paliatywna, Wydawnictwo Elsevier Urban&Partner, Wrocław 2012.

[9] Kinghorn S., Gaines S., Opieka Paliatywna, Wydawnictwo Elsevier Urban&Partner, Wrocław 2012.

the assessment of opinion and psychosocial and spiritual needs of the patient and his/her family.

Moreover, the patients are monitored every 4 or 12 hours, to exclude potential discomfort related to somatic, mental, and spiritual complaints, and the problems related to hygiene.

The postmortem care includes informing family members about the death of their relative and providing them with all necessary assistance. Information on the patient's death should be also provided to the team responsible for his/her primary care.

A Few Practical Advices…

What caregivers should not expect from a dying individual?

- that he/she will be brave
- that he/she will experience everything in silence
- that he/she will convert and would like to discuss the terminal problems
- that he/she will talk and ask questions
- that he/she will comfort the others.

What activities should be undertaken when contacting a dying individuals and his/her family:

- listening
- assistance (with a limit and distance defined by the patient himself/herself)
- answering when asked
- alleviating patient's suffering, including both the somatic and imperceptible suffering
- satisfying patient's needs, and motivating him/her to express his/her pent up needs.

What should not be practiced:

- instructing
- advising
- talking only to talk
- consolation that everything will improve

- deciding on behalf of the patient, believing that we know his/her needs and expectations better.

What should we be:

- sympathetic (spiritually rather than verbally and declaratively)
- empathic, sensitive
- careful
- patient
- self-controlled
- competent.

What should not we be:

- fearful
- official (cold)
- apodictic
- prudish
- intolerant
- impatient.

CONCLUSION

Professional career of a nurse comprises various stages associated with realizing her abilities with regards to life, dying, and death. The professionalism of a nurse can be manifested by her presence, care, assistance, and consolation; however, it is not always possible to get rid of the feeling of helplessness, lack of acceptance to passing away, and other strong emotions in view of patient's death.

Opinions, beliefs, and standards presented by people who take care for dying individuals (or assist them) do not legitimize them to make any decisions of behalf of their patients. Nothing can be imposed on the patient; moreover, he/she cannot perceive any mental or physical pressure to accept the other scenario than the one he/she has defined.

The care for dying individuals and their families requires active listening, and empathic co-experiencing and co-thinking. None expects any ready-to-use solutions or reliable patents.

We are well aware of our ignorance with regards to the moment of death. Nevertheless, despite our uniqueness and the end of our world, our death does not correspond to the end of life as a whole.

Good and calm passing away of their closest and beloved relative, free (or deprived) from pain and suffering, will be remembered well by the members of his/her family. Immediately after his/her death, also they will need help and support, including assistance in taking care for the body of their beloved one.

In: End-of-Life Care
Editors: Maria Rossi and Luiz Ortiz
ISBN: 978-1-62808-555-6

Chapter 6

SPIRITUALITY AT THE END-OF-LIFE

Beatriz Gil-Juliá* and Rafael Ballester-Arnal
Facultad de Ciencias de la Salud
Universitat Jaume I de Castellón, Spain

ABSTRACT

Facing death and the pain of the separation and the different losses is hard to bear for all those concerned. An important part of patient's discomfort does not come directly from the disease but from its subjective experience (Cassell, 1982). At this regard, physical or biological needs should be addressed, as well as social, emotional and spiritual ones.

Currently, it is recognized that spiritual factors may play an important role in the patient's serenity and suffering (Payás et al., 2008). For this reason this group of needs would have a great value, especially in the context of the end-of-life, where people cope with an array of difficulties and stressors, such as pain, feelings of uncertainty, and many changes at different levels because of the progression and irreversibility of the illness.

But what do we understand by spiritual needs? To define the concept of spirituality is not an easy task. Despite the fact that traditionally both terms, spirituality and religion, were practically inseparable, it is important not to confuse them. Spirituality is broader than religion, and an individual can be spiritual without being religious (Rowe & Allen,

* Corresponding author: Email: bgil@uji.es.

2004). This and other issues related to the spirituality at the end-of-life, such as the search for personal and psychological meaning, will be addressed in the present chapter.

INTRODUCTION

As people approach the end of their life multiple needs arise. It is a time of special vulnerability along which individuals struggle with the pain and suffering derived from the different losses they are facing. And one of the important healthcare professional's duties in this field is to ensure that this suffering is kept to a minimum.

At this regard, there is no doubt that pain and other physical symptoms are important issues to be managed but not the only ones. In order to provide the best care for those individuals whose life is drawing to a close, a holistic approach is required, including the attention to their physical, psychological, social and spiritual needs as the main organizations related to the end-of-life care avowed (National Consensus Project for Quality Palliative Care, 2009; National Institute for Clinical Excellence, 2004; Sanz, Gómez-Batiste, Gómez, & Núñez, 1993; World Health Organization, 2013).

It is worth noting that Dame Cecily Saunders, as early as the 60s, posing the foundations of palliative care, stated the importance of the spiritual dimension of the patient at the end-of-life (Saunders, 1990).

To the extent that it is widely recognized that spiritual factors may play a significant role in the patient's serenity and suffering (Payás et al., 2008), and therefore in their quality of life (Harrison et al., 2005), they need to be addressed and especially when people face a terminal diagnosis or even their own death.

RELIGION AND SPIRITUALITY

Defining the concept of religion and spirituality is often a difficult task. Despite the fact that traditionally both terms, spirituality and religion, were practically inseparable, they are becoming progressively distinct (Hill et al., 2000; Turner, Lukoff, Barnhouse, & Lu, 1995).

To better understand what it means to be religious or spiritual, clear definitions of these concepts are needed (Emmons & Paloutzian, 2003; Hill et al., 2000; Zinnbauer, Pargament, & Scott, 1999), and some of them are shown below.

Notwithstanding the lack of agreed definition of the meaning of spirituality, and as Tanyi (2002) stated in her review, different authors (Burkhardt, 1989; Emblen, 1992; Harrison, 1997; Reed, 1991; Relf 1997) include the following elements in their definitions of spirituality: transcendence, unfolding mystery, connectedness, meaning and purpose in life, higher power, and relationships. As well as, other researchers (La Pierre, 1994; Horsburgh, 1997; Walsh, 1999) considered that religion involves an organized entity with certain rituals, values, practices, and beliefs about God or a higher power.

Throughout the years, the approach to religion and spirituality has shifted. At this regard, it is worth noting in line with Zinnbauer et al. (1999) and as Schlehofer, Omoto and Adelman (2008) referred in their work that "religion may represent a set of organized practices established by tradition and conducted in a central place of worship, whereas spirituality is more personal. Religion holds a substantive focus on its practices, beliefs, and emotions, whereas spirituality is considered more functional, focusing on nature and being, and how beliefs, emotions, and practices relate to diverse life events like death, suffering, and injustice" (pp. 412).

Another conceptualization of religion and spirituality is proposed by Hill and colleagues (2000). These authors stated that, both religion and spirituality include two main components: a) the concept of the sacred (i.e., a perception of either some sense of ultimate reality or some divine being/object); and b) a search for the sacred (i.e., attempts to identify what is sacred, articulate at least to oneself what is identified, maintain or transform the sacred). Nevertheless, religion encompasses two additional components that spirituality does not: c) a search for the non-sacred (e.g., feelings of safety, hope, meaning, health or wellness); and d) a prescription of legitimate means and methods by which to search for the sacred (e.g., rituals or prescribed behaviors).

As noted, different definitions for the terms religion and spirituality exist though there not seems to be general consensus.

Summarizing, it is worth to bear in mind that spirituality is an inherent component of being human (Benjamin & Looby, 1998; Tanyi, 2000), is subjective, intangible, and multidimensional (Tanyi, 2000). Regardless of the two concepts, religion and spirituality, are often used interchangeably, they are different. Spirituality may be related to religion for certain individuals, but for others, it may not be (Tanyi, 2000). To this respect, spirituality is broader than religion, and an individual can be spiritual without being religious (Rowe & Allen, 2004).

Spiritual Needs

The importance of religion and spirituality when people cope with stressful situations, loss, and illness has been long accepted (Moadel et al., 1999; Narayanasamy, 2002; Sherwood, 2000). Spirituality may be also seen as a coping method in wellness and in a variety of diseases (Cooper-Effa, Blount, Kaslow, Rothenberg, & Eckman, 2001). Some authors, such as Puchalski and Romer (2000), even stated that "patients learn to cope with and understand their suffering through their spiritual beliefs, or the spiritual dimension of their lives" (pp. 129).

When analyzing the possible relationship between spirituality and health, spirituality is confirmed as a protective factor (Koenig, Larson & Weaver, 1998). Nevertheless, we cannot ignore that in some scenarios such as traumatic death, the resulting process may be accompanied by a significant spiritual struggle (Burke, Neimeyer, McDevitt-Murphy, Ippolito, & Roberts, 2011).

It is widely recognized that spiritual factors are elements that may contribute to the serenity or suffering of the patients (Payás et al., 2008), making this a special group of needs with great value at the end-of-life.

In line with this, Handzo and Koenig (2004) stated that "there is little disagreement any more in the healthcare community about whether spiritual care should be part of the treatment process. In many forums, the question has shifted to how spiritual care is to be provided and, more specifically, who should provide it" (pp. 1243).

All this emphasizes the significance of considering a holistic approach to patient well-being in the context of which, an important set of needs with own entity is becoming increasingly relevant, those called spiritual needs (Bayés & Borràs, 2005).

But what do we understand by spiritual needs? As mentioned previously, the terms spirituality and religion have been practically inseparable, but gradually the religious definition of spirituality has been substituted for a broader one and related to the psychological and personal search for meaning (Daaleman & VandeCreek, 2000). In words of Burnard (1988), these needs pertain to the search for meaning and purpose in life.

There is no doubt that any attempt to identify the main patient's spiritual needs is a hard endeavor. To shed light on this task different studies have been carried out. One of them (Emblen & Halstead, 1993) compared the responses of nurses, chaplains, and patients regarding the nature of spiritual needs. Spiritual needs were classified according to six categories:

1. Religious aspects, such as prayer and transcendence.
2. Experiences that are beyond earthly existence.
3. Affective feeling, including peace, comfort, and happiness.
4. Values, such as health, faith, and hope.
5. Communication, including talking, listening, and touching.
6. "Other" category, referring to such items as questions with death and voids.

Another important qualitative study was conducted by Taylor (2003) to describe the spiritual needs experienced by cancer patients. Her results identified 7 spiritual need categories:

1. The need to relate to an Ultimate Other.
2. The need for positivity, hope, and gratitude.
3. The need to give and receive love.
4. The need to review beliefs.
5. The need to have meaning.
6. The need related to religiosity.
7. The need to prepare for death.

And a more recent study worthy to consider is the one carried out by Galek, Flannelly, Vane & Galek (2005), whose analysis confirmed 7 constructs:

1. Love/belonging/respect: feeling unconditionally accepted; connecting to self and others; giving and receiving respect and love.
2. Divine: prayer; religious rituals; being part of a community; connecting with the divine.
3. Positivity/gratitude/hope/peace: peace; calm; sensing enjoyment in life; having hope; expressing humor and laughter.
4. Meaning and purpose: finding one's reason for living; finding meaning in one's personal history.
5. Morality and ethics: needing to live an ethical and responsible life.

6. Appreciation of beauty: connecting with beauty, nature, art, music, and the creative process.
7. Resolution/death: addressing concerns about life after death; gaining a deeper understanding of death and dying; coming to resolution about letting go; putting closure on life; offering forgiveness.

Of these, the most common construct was love and belonging, followed by religious needs.

In relation to the spiritual needs, it is of outstanding importance to consider that not only patients in this context experience these kind of needs but also their family (Taylor, 2003). In order to provide a total holistic care at the end-of-life, health care professionals should attend the relatives' spiritual needs in addition to the patients' ones, given the significant role played by the family in these circumstances.

And finally, when professionals are able to recognize what spiritual needs mean and whether they are present, there still left an important task: to identify when the individual is ready to discuss such affairs and concerns, that is to recognize the proper time for the patient to discuss them (VandeCreek, 1997).

Meeting the Spiritual Needs: Spiritual Care

The definition of spiritual care may be a bit uncertain. As Hanson et al. (2008) stated, "Spiritual care encompasses religious rituals and practices, as well as activities that comfort and support the person who is seriously ill as they search for meaning and for connection to what is infinite or transcendent" (pp. 907).

Each patient has his own response to the end-of-life. They have unique needs, included those spiritual ones. As part of the spiritual care offered, patients want healthcare professionals to show good qualities of humankind, and being encouraged by kind, compassionate, comforting and gentle care (Edwards, Pang, Shiu & Chan, 2010; Grant et al., 2004; Murray, Kendall, Boyd, Worth, & Benton, 2004).

In line with this, some authors as Barbero, Giró & Gomis (2008) affirmed that the healthcare professional should have different attitudes, which are not sufficient but necessary to provide a proper spiritual support. Those attitudes are the following:

- Hospitality: the person who hosts and offers support to the patient needs to feel comfortable with himself, without fear and with a certain peace of mind. In addition, the professional should facilitate the best place for the patient to explore their concerns and wounds without fear and with a kind of serenity. And this is only possible with the prior personal work of the professional in terms of his own spiritual life.
- The commitment to establish bonds, trust and show continuity and permanence. The key is not run away, do not ask the other "to undress in terms of exploring his worries and then do not help him to dress up". Likewise, the attitude of fidelity is compatible with assuming that the patient may choose another professional because patients fortunately speak with everyone, but listen only to those they choose.
- The professional must be able to sustain the patient in his pain during his inward journey, and then to allow him to go beyond his own self, if that is his choice. This may let the patient to find links beyond his own existence.
- Not only a detection attitude but also exploring, as well as not only waiting but also searching. That is an active approach to the spiritual dimension for two reasons. Firstly, it is important to stress that the goal in this field is to reduce the spiritual distress, if it does exist, as well as to promote the spiritual well-being. Secondly, the early detection and exploration of spiritual needs and resources allows us to take a necessary preventive dynamics, although initially there is no a specific request for support. Obviously, the exploration should be carried out with total prudence, respect and clearly no in an iatrogenic way. Moreover, it is necessary to bear in mind that the patient at one time could decide not to go deeper in his exploration, and our duty is to respect him absolutely, while also let him know that the professional is available whenever he decides to go forward.
- The healthcare professional has an important responsibility, which is related to his own care: to share his feelings with the working team in order to receive a proper supervision.

In addition to all these attitudes, professionals need both general and specialized *interventions* in order to alleviate patients suffering and enhance their spiritual aspects as they approach death. Palliative care, as a general frame of attention to these patients aims to improve quality of life, to enhance spiritual well-being, and to reduce suffering (Chochinov & Cann, 2005).

At this regard, there is clear evidence that traditional group psychotherapy interventions for cancer patients (one of the main contexts where to provide palliative care) are effective in improving quality of life and reducing psychological distress, anxiety, and depression, and in reducing physical symptoms. However, Breitbart (2002) in his review of existing psychotherapeutic interventions also notes that few cancer group psychotherapy intervention trials have focused specifically on existential or spiritual themes.

Some researchers have made important efforts to find intervention strategies to address spiritual needs. At this respect, Rousseau (2000) offers a practical guidance to alleviate spiritual distress in the dying patient, as follows: controlling physical symptoms; providing a supportive presence; encouraging life review to help the patient in recognizing purpose, value, and meaning; exploring guilt, remorse, forgiveness, and reconciliation; facilitating religious expression; reframing goals into short-term endeavors that can be accomplished; and focusing on the use of different practices, such as meditation, music, reading, poetry, and art that promote healing rather than cure.

On the other hand, Clark and Kissane (2002) offered another approach based on the construct named "demoralization". These authors recommend the adoption of demoralization syndrome as a relevant diagnostic entity in palliative care.

But what is understood by demoralization syndrome? Kissane, Clarke and Street (2001) defined this syndrome as "a psychiatric state in which hopelessness, helplessness, meaninglessness, and existential distress are the core phenomena" (pp. 13). And their treatment approach to alleviate the distress caused by this syndrome encompasses the following: provide continuity of care and active symptom management; explore attitudes toward hope and meaning in life; balance support for grief with promotion of hope; foster search for renewed purpose and role in life; use cognitive therapy to reframe negative beliefs; involve pastoral counseling for spiritual support; promote supportive relationships and use of volunteers; conduct family meetings to enhance their functioning; and review goals of care in multidisciplinary team meetings.

Finally, in an attempt to achieve a deeper understanding of specific spiritual care strategies we will outline two interesting initiatives.

The first one, the Meaning-Centered Group Psychotherapy by Breitbart and colleagues (Breitbart, 2002; Breitbart & Heller, 2003), which is based on the work of Viktor Frankl to address spiritual distress (in this case in the context of advanced cancer patients). The goal of this psychotherapy is to help participants to sustain or enhance a sense of meaning, peace, and purpose in their lives, even as they approach the end-of-life. This approach uses a combination of instruction, discussion, and experiential exercises in eight group sessions, with each session organized around a specific meaning-centered them. For therapists, the search for meaning is as a creative, individual, and active process, and therefore the patients are encouraged to be active participants in the group process.

The second one, called Dignity Therapy by Chochinov and colleagues (Chochinov, Hack, McClement, Harlos & Kristjanson, 2002) is empirically derived from their model of dignity towards the end-of-life. This therapy focuses on depression and suffering, along with on enhancing a sense of meaning, purpose and will to live in palliative care patients. As Chochinov and Cann (2005) refer, "the Dignity Therapy protocol offers an opportunity for patients to address aspects of life that they feel most proud of or that were most meaningful; the personal history that they most want remembered; or things that need to be said. This allows the patient to address grief-related issues, to offer comfort to soon-to-be bereft loved ones, or to provide instructions to friends and family" (pp. S111). Moreover, unlike other psychotherapies, this therapy is brief, can be done at the bed-side, and can affect both, patients and their relatives.

All this highlights the importance of a multidisciplinary approach, using appropriate spiritual coping strategies to the extent that they may enhance self-empowerment, leading to find meaning and purpose in illness, even at the end-of-life. This implies that holistic or total care addresses not only physical and psychological issues but also incorporates the facilitation of various spiritual coping strategies to safeguard the wholeness and integrity of patients (Baldacchino & Draper, 2001).

REFERENCES

Baldacchino, D. & Draper, P. (2001). Spiritual coping strategies: A review of the nursing research literature. *Journal of Advanced Nursing*, *34*, 833-841.

Barbero, J., Giró, R. M. & Gomis, C. (2008). El acompañamiento espiritual. In E. Benito, J. Barbero & A. Payás (Eds.), *El acompañamiento espiritual en cuidados paliativos* (109-141). Madrid: Arán Ediciones, S.L.

Bayés, R. & Borràs, F. X. (2005). ¿Qué son las necesidades espirituales?. *Medicina Paliativa*, *12*, 99-107.

Breitbart, W. (2002). Spirituality and meaning in supportive care: Spirituality- and meaning-centered group psychotherapy interventions in advanced cancer. *Supportive Care in Cancer*, *10*, 272-280.

Breitbart, W. & Heller, K. S. (2003). Reframing hope: Meaning-centered care for patients near the end-of-life. *Journal of Palliative Medicine*, *6*, 979-988.

Burke, L. A., Neimeyer, R. A., McDevitt-Murphy, M. E., Ippolito, M. R. & Roberts, J. M. (2011). Faith in the Wake of Homicide: Religious Coping and Bereavement Distress in an African American Sample. *International Journal for the Psychology of Religion*, *21*, 289-307.

Burkhardt, M. A. (1989). Spirituality: An analysis of the concept. *Holistic Nursing Practice*, *3*, 69-77.

Burnard, P. (1988). The spiritual needs of atheists and agnostics. *Professional Nurse*, *4*, 130-132.

Cassel, E. J. (1982). The nature of suffering and the goals of medicine. *The New England Journal of Medicine*, *306*, 639-645.

Chochinov, H. M. & Cann, B. J. (2005). Interventions to enhance the Spiritual Aspects of Dying. *Journal of Palliative Medicine*, *8*, S103-S115.

Chochinov, H. M., Hack, T., McClement, S., Harlos, M. & Kristjanson, L. (2002). Dignity in the terminally ill: An empirical model. *Social Science and Medicine*, *54*, 433-443.

Clarke, D. M. & Kissane, D. W. (2002). Demoralization: Its phenomenology and importance. *Australian and New Zealand Journal of Psychiatry*, *36*, 733-742.

Cooper-Effa M., Blount, W., Kaslow, N., Rothenberg, R. & Eckman, J. (2001). Role of spirituality in patients with sickle cell disease. *Journal of the American board of family medicine*, *14*, 116-122.

Edwards, A., Pang, N., Shiu, V. & Chan, C. (2010). The understanding of spirituality and the potential role of spiritual care in end-of-life and palliative care: a meta-study of qualitative research. *Palliative Medicine*, *24*, 753-770.

Emblen, J. D. (1992). Religion and spirituality defined according to current use in nursing literature. *Journal of Professional Nursing*, *8*, 41-47.

Emblen, J. D. & Halstead, L. (1993). Spiritual needs and interventions: comparing the views of patients, nurses, and chaplains. *Clinical Nurse Specialist*, *7*, 175-182.

Emmons, R. A. & Paloutzian, R. F. (2003). The psychology of religion. *Annual Review of Psychology*, *54*, 377-402.

Galek, K., Flannelly, K. J., Vane, A. & Galek, L. M. (2005). Assessing a Patient's Spiritual Needs. A Comprehensive Instrument. *Holistic Nursing Practice*, *19*, 62-69.

Grant, E., Murray, S. A., Kendall, M., Boyd, K., Tilley, S. & Ryan, D. (2004). Spiritual issues and needs: perspectives from patients with advanced cancer and nonmalignant disease. A qualitative study. *Palliative & Support Care*, *2*, 371-378.

Handzo, G. & Koenig, H. G. (2004). Spiritual care: whose job is it anyway? *Southern Medical Journal*, *97*, 1242-1244.

Hanson, L. C., Dobbs, D., Usher, B. M., Williams, S., Rawlings, J., & Daaleman, T. P. (2008). Providers and types of spiritual care experienced during serious illness. *Journal of Palliative Medicine*, *11*, 907-914.

Harrison, M. O., Edwards, C. L., Koenig, H. G., Bosworth, H. B., Decastro, L. & Wood, M. (2005). Religiosity/Spirituality and Pain in Patients With Sickle Cell Disease. *Journal of Nervous & Mental Disease*, *193*, 250-257.

Harrison, R. L. (1997). Spirituality and hope: nursing implications for people with HIV disease. *Holistic Nursing Practice*, *12*, 9-16.

Hill, P. C., Pargament, K. I., Hood, R. W., McCullough, M. E., Swyers, J. P., Larson, D. B. & Zinnbauer, B. J. (2000). Conceptualizing religion and spirituality: Points of commonality, points of departure. *Journal for the Theory of Social Behaviour*, *30*, 51-77.

Horsburgh, M. (1997). Towards an inclusive spirituality: wholeness, interdependence and waiting. *Disability and Rehabilitation*, *19*, 398-406.

Kissane, D. W., Clarke, D. M. & Street, A. F. (2001). Demoralization syndrome—a relevant psychiatric diagnosis for palliative care. *Journal of Palliative Care*, *17*, 12-21.

Koenig, H. G., Larson, D. B. & Weaver, A. J. (1998). Research on religion and serious mental illness. *New Directions for Mental Health Services*, *80*, 81-95.

LaPierre, L. (1994). A model for describing spirituality. *Journal of Religion and Health*, *33*, 153-161.

Moadel, A., Morgan, C., Fatone, A., Grennan, J., Carter, J., Laruffa, G., Skummy, A. & Dutcher, J. (1999). Seeking meaning and hope: self-reported spiritual and existential needs among an ethnically-diverse cancer patient population. *Psycho-Oncology*, *8*, 378-385.

Murray, S. A., Kendall, M., Boyd, K., Worth, A. & Benton, T. F. (2004). Exploring the spiritual needs of people dying of lung cancer or heart failure: a prospective qualitative interview study of patients and their carers. *Palliative Medicine*, *18*, 39-45.

Narayanasamy, A. (2002). Spiritual coping mechanisms in chronically ill patients. *British Journal of Nursing*, *11*, 1461-1470.

National Consensus Project for Quality Palliative Care. (2009). Clinical practice guidelines for quality palliative care. http://www.nationalconsensusproject.org/guideline.pdf. (accessed 15 March 2008).

National Institute for Clinical Excellence. (2004). *Improving supportive and palliative care for adults with cancer*. London: NICE.

Payás, A., Barbero, J., Bayés, R., Benito, E., Giró, R. M., Maté, J., Rodeles, R. Y. & Tomás, C. M. (2008). ¿Cómo perciben los profesionales de paliativos las necesidades espirituales del paciente al final de la vida?. *Medicina Paliativa*, *15*, 225-237.

Puchalski, C. M. & Romer, A. L. (2000). Taking a spiritual history allows clinicians to understand patients more fully. *Journal of Palliative Medicine*, *3*, 129-137.

Reed, P. G. (1991). Spirituality and mental health in older adults: extant knowledge for nursing. *Family and Community Health*, *14*, 14-25.

Relf, M. V. (1997). Illuminating meaning and transforming issues of spirituality in HIV disease and Aids: an application of Parse's theory of human being. *Holistic Nursing Practice*, *12*, 1-8.

Rousseau, P. (2000). Spirituality and the dying patient. *Journal of Clinical Oncology*, *18*, 2000-2002.

Rowe, M. M. & Allen, R. G. (2004). Spirituality as a means of coping with chronic illness. *American Journal of Health Studies*, *19*, 62-67.

Sanz, J., Gómez-Batiste, X., Gómez, M. & Núñez, J. M. (1993).*Cuidados paliativos: recomendaciones de la Sociedad Española de Cuidados Paliativos (SECPAL)*. Madrid: Ministerio de Sanidad y Consumo.

Saunders, C. (1990). *Hospice and palliative care*. Londres: Arnold.

Schlehofer, M. M., Omoto, A. M. & Adelman, J. R. (2008). How do "Religion" and "Spirituality" Differ? Lay Definitions Among Older Adults. *Journal for the Scientific Study of Religion*, *47*, 411-425.

Sherwood, G. D. (2000). The power of nurse-client encounters: interpreting spiritual themes. *Journal of Holistic Nursing*, *18*, 159-175.

Tanyi, R. A. (2002). Towards clarification of the meaning of spirituality. *Journal of Advanced Nursing*, *39*, 500-509.

Taylor, E. J. (2003). Spiritual needs of patients with cancer and family caregivers. *Cancer Nursing*, *26*, 260-266.

Turner, R. P., Lukoff, D., Barnhouse, R. T. & Lu, F. G. (1995). Religious or spiritual problem: A culturally sensitive diagnostic category in the DSM-IV. *Journal of Nervous and Mental Disease*, *183*, 435-444.

VandeCreek, L. (1997). Collaboration between nurses and chaplains for Spiritual Caregiving. *Seminars in Oncology Nursing*, *13*, 279-280.

Walsh, F. (1999). Religion and spirituality: wellspring for healing and resilience. In F. Walsh (Ed.), *Spiritual Resources in Family Therapy* (3-27). New York: Guilford Publications.

World Health Organization. (2013). WHO definition of palliative care. http://www.who.int/cancer/palliative/definition/en/ (accessed 12 March 2013).

Zinnbauer, B. J., Pargament, K. I. & Scott, A. B. (1999). The emerging meanings of religiousness and spirituality: Problems and prospects. *Journal of Personality*, *67*, 889-919.

In: End-of-Life Care
Editors: Maria Rossi and Luiz Ortiz
ISBN: 978-1-62808-555-6

Chapter 7

CHALLENGES OF PROMOTING END-OF-LIFE CARE IN RESIDENTIAL CARE HOMES IN HONG KONG

***Helen Y. L. Chan*[*1], *Samantha M. C. Pang and Edward M. F. Leung*[2]**

[1]The Nethersole School of Nursing, Faculty of Medicine, The Chinese University of Hong Kong
[2]School of Nursing, The Hong Kong Polytechnic University
[3]United Christian Hospital, Hong Kong, Hong Kong Association of Gerontology

ABSTRACT

Growing attention is being paid to the healthcare needs of older people who live with advanced diseases or disabilities. Studies have shown that frail older people share similar concerns and needs as patients who have terminal diseases. End-of-life care should therefore be extended to older people who are experiencing a progressive worsening of their health and functional ability. In Hong Kong, older people living in residential care homes are relatively frailer because moving to a long-term care setting is usually the last resort when their substantial care needs cannot be met at home. Hence, a residential care home is an optimal place for promoting end-of-life care. However, end-of-life care

* Email: helencyl@cuhk.edu.hk.

has yet to be systematically integrated into the care practice in this setting. This chapter will discuss three major challenges in promoting end-of-life care in residential care homes for older people: (1) whether Chinese older people are willing to openly talk about issues of death and dying; (2) whether family members and healthcare providers are willing to support end-of-life care provision; and (3) whether end-of-life care development is facilitated in the community.

BACKGROUND

Healthcare service in Hong Kong is renowned for its affordability, accessibility and high quality (Food and Health Bureau, 2008). Over the last few decades highly complex and sophisticated care has changed the leading cause of death from acute health problems to those of a chronic nature. The number of people aged 65 and above has recently increased nearly twofold, from 6.6% in 1981 to 13.3% in 2011 (Census and Statistics Department, 2012). Yet, more than two-thirds of them have at least one chronic disease and 22.7% of them suffer from three or more types of co-morbidity (Census and Statistics Department, 2009). Health decline is anticipated as these diseases progress to advanced stages. To these older people, merely focusing the goal of medicine on life-saving would seem to be of limited benefits; this is because it fails to address their major needs and concerns during their final years of life (Chan & Pang, 2007, Luk, Liu, Ng, Lui, Beh & Chan, 2010). End-of-life care, which is an integral part of palliative care, has therefore emerged as a tenet to optimize physical, psychosocial and spiritual well-being during the final phase of life (End of Life Care Strategy, 2008). In line with this, a guide to good nursing practice on end-of-life care has been formulated by the Nursing Council of Hong Kong (2006), and it reaffirms the importance of facilitating a dignified and peaceful closure of life in patients who have a grave prognosis.

The need for end-of-life care has been increasingly recognized across the world. A benchmarking exercise in end-of-life care provision was conducted by the Economist Intelligence Unit (EIU) in 2010. A "Quality of Death" Index, which comprises 24 indicators related to the quality of end-of-life care, the availability of end-of-life care, the end-of-life healthcare environment and the cost, was derived. Among the 40 regions included in the exercise, Hong Kong was generally ranked twentieth, and that it is behind Asian regions such as Taiwan and Singapore (EIU, 2010). Hong Kong's score was particularly poor in the basic end-of-life healthcare environment, being thirty-first in this category. The poor scoring therein may be partly explained in terms of limited funding and resources to improve end-of-life care development, and the lack of recognition in the government healthcare policy in this area, yet the underlying reasons for these are probably due to the predominant life preservation culture in the practice of medicine and healthcare.

A Culture of Death Denial

Increased life expectancy has been recognized as one of the greatest triumphs of modern health care development; death is therefore viewed as a failure of medicine rather than a natural process in life. Due to death denial culture, a healthcare team would rarely initiate a discussion to elicit the patients' end-of-life care needs and preferences, and neither would the patients plan ahead for their future care. The relevant decision-making process is often deferred until a health crisis occurs.

Against such a background, family members and health professionals are usually in a difficult position if they are required to make decisions for the patients. Patients might no longer be able to participate in the decision-making process at times of severe ill health. Although family members do not have legal status in surrogate decision-making in Hong Kong, the healthcare team needs to weigh their choices seriously. Family members and health professionals then work together to arrive at a consensus regarding the care plan (Hospital Authority, 2002, Medical Council, 2009). The problems are that they usually do not know the patients' care wishes, and it would be emotionally overwhelming for them to balance the benefits and burdens of different treatment options at that critical moment. Literature shows that Chinese family members tend to choose aggressive treatment for patients based on unrealistic expectations or filial obligation (Kwok, Twinn & Yan, 2007, Tang, Lam & Chiu, 2007). Due to the medicalization of death, health professionals may also perceive the pressure to perform curative treatment. Hence, both family members and the healthcare team tend to regard saving life as their absolute moral duty.

The above shows that the avoidance approach towards end-of-life care planning in a death denial culture results in a lose–lose situation. The lack of advance planning deprives patients of their right to self-determination in the end-of-life care decision-making process, and this might result in the situation that during their last days patients have to receive treatment and care that they do not wish to receive. Most of the patients who have terminal or chronic diseases experience recurrent hospitalization in the last phase of life. The lack of communication also gives rise to stress, anxiety and depression among family members, and it also causes disputes between family members and the healthcare team over care decisions for patients in their final stage of life.

CHALLENGES FOR END-OF-LIFE CARE

The death denial culture largely accounts for the difficulties of end-of-life care development in Hong Kong, but is such a culture formed just because death is a taboo subject in Chinese society? The Quality of Death Index shows that Hong Kong has a poor rating in multiple aspects related to end-of-life care provision. This section therefore aims to identify the major challenges at individual, caregiver, and community level that hinder the promotion of end-of-life care in residential care homes in Hong Kong.

Individual Level

Death and dying have traditionally been regarded as taboo in Chinese culture (EIU, 2010). Older people might therefore be presumed to be more conservative in discussing such sensitive issues. On the contrary, several studies conducted in residential care homes and hospitals found that many older people would like to be informed of their diagnosis and prognosis, and that they appreciate opportunities to express their views on their end-of-life care and to participate in their care planning (Chan & Pang, 2007; Chu et al., 2011, Mok, Ting & Lau, 2010). This finding contradicts the notion that the issues of death and dying are cultural taboos among older Chinese people.

Involving older people in end-of-life care planning would, therefore, be an initial step in promoting end-of-life care. Nevertheless, most of them were not aware that they have the right to make choices in healthcare decisions, and they simply trusted the physicians to make decisions in their best interests. Chan and Pang (2010) found that the advance care planning process allows older people to reflect on their personal values and beliefs and it empowers them to share their views towards end-of-life care. The planning process also encourages them to communicate their care wishes openly with their significant others.

The study further revealed the diverse opinions among Chinese older people towards end-of-life care decision-making (Chan & Pang, 2011). Five approaches were identified among the 42 frail residents who underwent advance care planning, as shown in Figure 1, namely: holding onto life; weighing benefits; planning ahead; avoiding; and deferral (Chan & Pang, 2011).

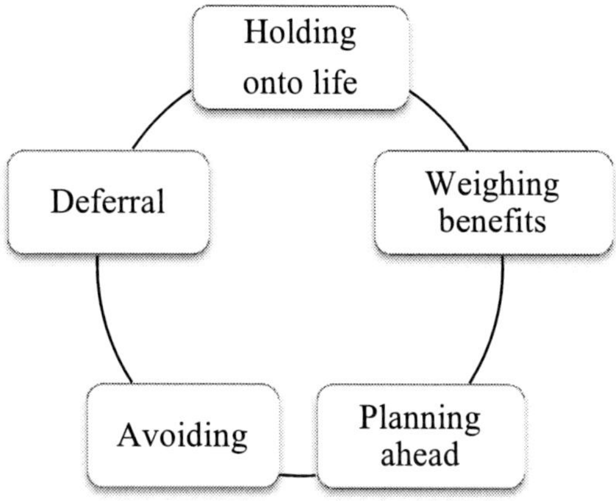

Figure 1. Different approaches towards end-of-life care decision making.

A lack of awareness towards their rights in healthcare decision-making was apparent among the participants. A considerable number of residents had not contemplated the issues seriously before the study because they were not aware of their role in the decision-making process. They were then empowered by the advance care planning process and were able to indicate their end-of-life care wishes, no matter what their wishes were, to try every means to save life, as in the holding-onto-life approach or to forgo treatment that they considered futile, as in the weighing-benefits approach. Their involvement can be improved by heightening their awareness towards their right to self-determination through an advance care planning programme.

On the contrary, some participants had planned well ahead for their future care even before the advance care planning programme. The care planning process thus provided a platform for them to share their care wishes. The above shows that the presumption that Chinese older people are reluctant to discuss end-of-life care issues is fallacious. The successful experience in end-of-life care in Taiwan and Singapore also evidences that Chinese culture is not the major impediment to end-of-life care development (EIU, 2010).

Their readiness for end-of-life care decision-making has to be assessed on an individual basis. The study (Chan & Pang 2011) also revealed that some older people avoided thinking about end-of-life care because of death anxiety. Some expressed a sense of powerlessness over their health conditions and they wanted to delegate the decision-making to their family members or healthcare team. However, it is premature to conclude that introducing the concept of advance care planning to these residents would be inappropriate. Prospective longitudinal study is needed to examine whether older people would change their decisions over time.

Caregiver Level

With filial piety as a major core value in Chinese culture, family members are often expected to share the care responsibilities of providing functional and emotional support to older family members. The perceived filial obligations of these informal caregivers sometimes hinder them from making substitute judgements for older members of their family. This is not only because it is difficult for family members to predict the care wishes of older people who have moved into residential care homes; this means that they are usually more emotionally distant. More often the struggles arise from the sense of indebtedness among the family members, and as such they are reluctant to forgo any hope of recovery. This gives rise to the phenomenon that younger family members are more unwilling to openly talk about death and dying issues than the older members (Chan & Pang, 2010). Family members often are less prepared to make the difficult decisions. Because forgoing treatment might be misunderstood in the family and in the culture, they may err towards life preservation at all costs so as to avoid conflicts or ensuing feelings of guilt (Chan, Ho, Leung, Chochinov, Neimeyer, Pang, & Tse, 2012).

Compared to family members, healthcare providers should have a better understanding of the limitations of the current curative treatments and how the patients' concerns can be better addressed by end-of-life care. However, several studies have revealed that capacity building for healthcare providers with regard to end-of-life care is inadequate. A survey study has reported that frontline staff in residential care homes perceive that they lack both the knowledge and the ability to deliver end-of-life care to the residents (Chan, Leung, Ng & Pang, 2012). Even nurses in an oncology setting, who are the key to quality care for the terminally ill, consider themselves as not being adequately prepared to give the necessary care provision (Chan, Lee & Chan, 2012).

Healthcare providers have frequent interactions with clients. Their attitudes and perceptions towards end-of-life care have great impact on the culture of promoting end-of-life care. This highlights the importance of building the capacity for end-of-life care in the frontline staff of healthcare settings, including those in residential care homes. Several non-government organizations and professional bodies, such as the Society for the Promotion of Hospice Care (SPHC), the Hong Kong Association of Gerontology (HKAG), have provided relevant training to frontline staff working in residential care homes (SPHC, 2013, HKAG, 2013). However, such training has not been incorporated into the regular training. The home staff who work in those residential care homes where the importance of end-of-life care for older people is not realized, might therefore not be aware of their role in end-of-life care provision. This echoes with the EIU's study (2010) that the basic end-of-life healthcare environments in Hong Kong are not properly prepared.

While staff training in end-of-life care can be improved by increasing resources, the question of how to measure the quality of end-of-life care, particularly in the psychosocial and spiritual aspects, can hardly be answered directly. Conventional clinical outcomes, such as survival rate, healthcare utilization and cost-effectiveness analysis, seem incommensurable for evaluating end-of-life care. The Quality of Death Index evaluated the care quality in terms of public awareness, training availability, pain control, and doctor–patient transparency (EIU, 2010). These are important indicators, but sometimes they may not reflect the care experience of the clients. It is noticeable from the literature that consensus on outcome measures for end-of-life care has not yet been reached among researchers and clinicians. Due to different objectives, some studies used quality of life as the care outcome, whereas others focused on the completion rate of advance directives and the level of decisional conflicts after the study. So, should end-of-life care planning be considered as a failure if the quality of life has not been significantly improved during the last phase of life? What if the patients express inconsistent care wishes, or if they fail to indicate their care wishes during the process? The problem of assessment is more apparent if the patients are mentally incompetent. All these invite criticism on how end-of-life care can be evaluated.

Community Level

In Hong Kong, the development of end-of-life care is often not on the agenda of policy-makers. There is neither a clear policy nor a timeline on improving its quality and promoting public awareness towards the patients' right to self-determination in end-of-life care (Luk et al., 2011). For example, the Law Reform Commission of Hong Kong (2006) concluded from a public consultation on Substitute Decision-making and Advance Directives in relation to Medical Treatment that the subject remains a taboo in the culture and more public education is needed in the community, but again these works for promoting public awareness have been left to non-government organizations and professional bodies.

The death-denying culture and the lack of a supportive environment to end-of-life care development in residential care homes also add difficulties to the hope of dying in place. In Hong Kong, a considerable number of residents wish to die in their care homes accompanied by their family members but most of them are sent to hospital in their last days (Chu et al., 2011, Luk et al., 2011). Not only because the home staff were not ready to take care of dying residents, there was also difficulty in the care home reserving a private and spacious room for the dying resident and their family members inside its premise. In the death-denying culture, letting a resident pass away in the care home will likely have a significant psychological impact both on the co-residents and on the neighbours in the wider community (Leung, 2011).

Another major concern is about the legal liability of the care home in the event of a resident passing away under its care (Leung, 2011). The current law requires residential care homes to report each inhouse death to the police, and it also requires the Coroner to investigate the cause of the death. For this reason, the dead body has to be sent to the public mortuary rather than directly to the funeral home. This explains why residents who obviously have a grave prognosis have to be sent to hospital for death pronouncement during their last hours (Luk et al., 2011). It can be seen that because the concept of promoting end-of-life care in residential care homes has not been considered in the current policy and law, procedures which are intended to protect the residents are now becoming a barrier to a peaceful death.

WAY FORWARD

The development of end-of-life care in residential care homes in Hong Kong is now seriously lagging, in part due to the death-denying culture. Such a culture prevails not because the older people are reluctant to talk about death and dying issues, but because the family members, healthcare providers and the policy-makers have yet to orchestrate their efforts in integrating palliative care to the healthcare system. A concerted effort is therefore needed to promote end-of-life care. At the individual level, it is important to engage the older people and their family members in advance planning for end-of-life care so as to empower the older people to express their care wishes and let their family members understand their views. At the caregiver level, capacity building related to end-of-life care is needed for healthcare providers including residential care homes and hospital for availability and access to quality palliative care at the end-of-life in accordance to older people's preferences.

At present, palliative care is missing from Hong Kong's public health policy. The Strategic Framework for Prevention and Control of Non-communicable Diseases, formulated by the Department of Health (2008), has highlighted the importance of achieving a reduction in premature deaths, but makes no mention of the role of palliative care. As the United Nations (2011) have asked member states to include palliative care as an integral part of national policies for addressing non-communicable disease challenges, we envisage that Hong Kong will follow the initiative taken by other countries in developing policies to make palliative care available to the public at large. The mainstream view of the professional associations of Hong Kong holds that palliative care can foster comfort and dignity. Recent studies consistently show that Hong Kong as a community should be ready to take a more proactive step in promoting advance directives as well as preparing health professionals' readiness and competencies in engaging patients and their family members in advance care planning. The challenge for the future is how to develop policies and a care service model that includes palliative care as an integral part of the health and social care systems.

REFERENCES

Census and Statistics Department. (2009). Thematic household survey report no. 40: Socio-demographic profile, health status and self-care capability of older persons. Hong Kong SAR Government.

Census and Statistics Department. (2012). Demographic trends in Hong Kong (1981 – 2011). Hong Kong SAR Government.

Chan, C.L.W., Ho, A.H.Y., Leung, P.P.Y., Chochinov, H.M., Neimeyer, R.A., Pang, S.M.C., & Tse, D.M.W. (2012). The blessings and the curses of filial piety on dignity at the end of life: Lived experience of Hong Kong Chinese adult children caregivers. Journal of Ethnic & Cultural Diversity in Social Work, 21, 277–296.

Chan, H.Y.L., & Pang, S.M.C. (2011). Readiness of Chinese frail old age home residents to end-of-life care decision making. Journal of Clinical Nursing, 20, 1454-1461.

Chan, H.Y.L., & Pang, S.M.C. (2010). Let Me Talk – an advance care planning programme for frail nursing home residents. Journal of Clinical Nursing, 19, 3073-3084.

Chan, H. Y. L., & Pang, S. M. C. (2007). Quality of life concerns and end-of-life care preferences of aged persons in long-term care facilities. Journal of Clinical Nursing, 16, 2158-2166.

Chan, H.Y.L., Lee, L.H., & Chan, C.W.H. (2012). The perceptions and experiences of nurses and bereaved families towards bereavement care in an oncology unit. Supportive Care in Cancer, DOI: 10.1007/s00520-012-1692-4

Chan, H.Y.L., Leung, E.M.F., Ng, E.Y.K. & Pang, S.M.C. (2012). Palliative care in residential care homes for the elderly program: impacts on staffs' willingness, perceived competence and resilience. Proceedings of Nineteenth Annual Congress of Gerontology, 2012.

Chu, L.W., Luk, J.K., Hui, E., Chiu, P.K., Chan, C.S., Kwan, F., Kwok, F., Lee, D. & Woo, J. (2011). Advance directive and end-of-life care preferences among Chinese nursing home residents in Hong Kong. Journal of American Medical Director Association, 12(2), 143-152.

Department of Health (2008). Promoting health in Hong Kong; A strategic framework for prevention and control of non-communicable diseases. The Hong Kong SAR Government.

Economist Intelligence Unit (EIU). (2010). The quality of death: Ranking end-of-life care across the world. Lien Foundation.

End of Life Care Strategy. (2008). Promoting high quality care for all adults at the end of life. UK Department of Health.

Food and Health Bureau. (2008). Your health your life: Healthcare reform consultation document. Hong Kong SAR Government.

Hong Kong Association of Gerontology. (2013). Training courses. Retrieved from http://hkag.org/Courses.htm

Hospital Authority. (2002). HA guidelines on life-sustaining treatment in the terminally ill. Hospital Authority Clinical Ethics Committee.

Kwok, T., Twinn, S., & Yan, E. (2007). The attitudes of Chinese family caregivers of older people with dementia towards life sustaining treatments. Journal of Advanced Nursing, 58, 256-262.

Law Reform Commission of Hong Kong. (2006). Report on substitute decision-making and advance directives in relation to medical treatment. Hong Kong SAR Government.

Leung, E.M.F. (2011). End of life care issues in Chinese population – Implications for practice. Presented at the Canadian Geriatrics Society on End of Life Care in Long Term Care Settings, 2011.

Luk, J.K.H., Liu, A., Ng, W.C., Lui, B., Beh, P., & Chan, F.H.W. (2010). End-of-life care: Towards a more dignified dying process in residential care homes for the elderly. Hong Kong Medical Journal, 16(3), 235-236.

Luk, J.K.H., Liu, A., Ng, W.C., Beh, P., & Chan, F.H.W. (2011). End-of-life care in Hong Kong. Asian Journal of Gerontology and Geriatrics, 6, 103-106.

Medical Council of Hong Kong. (2009) Code of professional conduct for the guidance of registered of medical practitioners. Hong Kong.

Mok, E., Ting, F.H., & Lau, K.P. (2010). Advance directive and life-sustaining treatment: informed attitudes of Hong Kong Chinese elders with chronic disease. Journal of Nursing and Healthcare of Chronic Illness, 2, 313-319.

Nursing Council of Hong Kong. (2002) Code of professional conduct and code of ethics for nurses in Hong Kong. Hong Kong.

Nursing Council of Hong Kong. (2006). Guide to good nursing practice: End-of-life care.

Society for the Promotion of Hospice Care. (2013). End of life care training programme for health care workers. Retrieved from http://www2.hospicecare.org.hk/our-work/training/for-health-professionals/

Tang, C.S.H., Lam, L.C.W., & Chiu, H.F.K. (2007). Attitudes of end-of-life decisions: A survey of elderly Chinese with dementia and their carers. Asian Journal of Gerontology and Geriatrics, 2, 119-125.

United Nations. (2011). Political declaration of the high-level meeting of the General Assembly on the prevention and control of non-communicable diseases. Retrieved from http://www.un.org/en/ga/ncdmeeting2011/documents.shtml

In: End-of-Life Care
Editors: Maria Rossi and Luiz Ortiz
ISBN: 978-1-62808-555-6

Expert Commentary

ARE VETERINARIANS KINDER THAN PHYSICIANS AT END-OF-LIFE? IS PAWSPICE KINDER THAN HOSPICE? A VETERINARY ONCOLOGIST'S INTERPROFESSIONAL CROSSOVER PERSPECTIVE OF EUTHANASIA FOR TERMINAL PATIENTS

Alice Villalobos[*]
The Society for Veterinary Medial Ethics and The American Association of Human-Animal Bond Veterinarians, Pawspice and Animal Oncology Consultation Service, Hermosa Beach & Woodland Hills, California, US

INTRODUCTION

This discussion is an expert commentary on why and how society seems to maintain a dual ethic on standards for quality of life at the end-of-life between animal vs. human patients. Due to the cherished value of the human-animal bond in society, veterinary medical practitioners adopted the pediatrician model. The unique difference between a small animal practitioner's vs. a pediatrician's end-of-life approach is that their companion animal patients are considered geriatric babies!

[*] Corresponding author: www.pawspice.com, pawspice@yahoo.com.

This author is a practicing veterinary oncologist with 40 plus years of experience serving clients and their animal cancer patients with Pawspice, a practice which simultaneously embraces both palliative and standard care. When quality of life (QoL) declines to the point where the patient can no longer enjoy life, clients are compassionately counseled to consider the gift of humane euthanasia for their beloved pets. (Villalobos) When pet owners fail to recognize the relentless suffering and frustration of their dying companion animals, the attending veterinary medical staff endures distress which may result in a nagging moral stress that makes them more prone to compassion fatigue. Veterinarians serve society as healers. They have the oath and responsibility of compassionately preventing suffering in their patients. This includes preventing the misery and anguish of being forced to endure a prolonged or bad death. (Rollin)

Human longing for euthanasia is especially fulminate when the body is in relentless decline yet being kept in suspension to scientifically defy death. This is accomplished very well via modern medicine and life supportive care in ICU's and skilled nursing homes. The science ideology that death can and should be defeated, no matter the cost, is standard of practice for a large majority of physicians. This unique thinking is very American. It is encouraged by the innovative for-profit medical marketplace which has not yet defeated the inevitability of death. Physician detachment from death is unsustainable and imposes great emotional stress on patients and their families and a foreboding expense on the health care system for baby boomers.

Double Standard for Animal vs. Human Death

Society condones and encourages euthanasia for terminal animals to provide relief and prevent futile suffering. This allows a peaceful and painless passage for dying companion animal patients and emotional and financial relief for their devoted caregivers. Many people openly grieve more for their beloved companion animals than for their relatives. (Kaplan) This is because that particular animal was their joy, their social lubricant, the subject of their daily care giving, walking, hiking, reading, watching TV and living with unconditional love. The feelings of pet loss and bereavement are not much different than the loss and emotional grief suffered by those who have lost children or spouses whom they loved deeply and greatly cared for.

Bioethicist, Jessica Pierce, Ph.D. asks in *Psychology Today*, Why is euthanasia almost always considered the compassionate end point for our

animals, but not for our human companions? (Pierce) http://www.psychology today.com/experts/jessica-pierce-phd

Table 1. Quality of Life Scale

Quality of Life Scale (The HHHHHMM QoL Scale)	
Pet caregivers can use this Quality of Life Scale to determine the success of Pawspice care. Score patients using a scale of: 0 to 10 (0 being the worst condition and 10 being ideal).	
Score	**Criterion**
0-10	**HURT** - Adequate pain control & breathing ability are of top concern. If the pet can't breathe properly, nothing else matters. This criterion outweighs all others! Is oxygen supplementation necessary? Is the pet's pain well managed?
0-10	**HUNGER** - Is the pet eating enough? Does hand feeding help? Does the pet need a feeding tube?
0-10	**HYDRATION** - Is the pet dehydrated? For patients not drinking enough, use subcutaneous fluids daily to supplement fluid intake.
0-10	**HYGIENE** - The pet should be brushed and cleaned, particularly after eliminations. Avoid pressure sores with soft bedding and keep all wounds clean.
0-10	**HAPPINESS** - Does the pet express joy and interest? Is the pet responsive to family, toys, etc.? Is the pet depressed, lonely, anxious, bored or afraid? Can the pet's bed be moved to be close to family activities?
0-10	**MOBILITY** - Can the pet get up without assistance? Does the pet need human or mechanical help (e.g., a cart)? Does the dog feel like going for a walk? Is the pet having seizures or stumbling? (Some carers feel that euthanasia is preferable to amputation, but an animal with limited mobility yet still alert and responsive, can have a good quality of life as long as the family is committed to helping their pet.)
0-10	**MORE GOOD DAYS THAN BAD** - When bad days outnumber good days, quality of life might be too compromised. When a healthy human-animal bond is no longer possible, the carers must be made aware that the end is near. The decision for euthanasia needs to be made if the pet is suffering. It is ideal when a pet's death comes peacefully and painlessly at home.
***TOTAL**	*A total over 35 points represents acceptable life quality to continue with pet hospice (Pawspice).

Original concept, *Oncology Outlook*, by Dr. Alice Villalobos, *Quality of Life Scale Helps Make Final Call*, VPN, 09/2004; formatted for *Canine and Feline Geriatric Oncology: Honoring the Human-Animal Bond*, Blackwell Publishing, 2007. Adapted for: AVMA, NAVC, VSIPP, IVAPM & AAFP Hospice Guidelines, 2013 SVME online Basic Veterinary Medical Ethics Course, *Canine and Feline Anesthesia, Consultations in Feline Medicine*, Nova Publications, with permission.

Quality of Life Should Include Happiness

This author created a special user friendly quality of life scale that measures seven basic criteria which veterinarians accept as universal welfare for animals. The seven criteria were condensed into an easily recalled acronym of five H's: Hurt, Hunger, Hydration, Hygiene, Happiness and two M's: Mobility and More good days than bad days. This scale is called the "HHHHHMM" Quality of Life Scale, wherein one pronounces the acronym like the word, hum. This scale went viral in the veterinary community and it has helped tens of thousands of pet owners worldwide identify if they were properly caring for their end-of-life companion animal. The QoL Scale helps the veterinary team partner with pet owners in the difficult decision making process of whether to continue their pet's Pawspice or if it is appropriate to provide the gift of euthanasia. Many people have used this scale in evaluating the status quo of their elderly and dying family members because QoL is not just the absence of disease and pain. See Table 1. (Villalobos)

What Physicians Want for Themselves

Health care professionals are committed to helping their patients get the best outcome under the given circumstances of their disease conditions and co morbidities. Society readily condones the gift of euthanasia to relieve and prevent the relentless and futile suffering of animals. This reflects the good shepherd role that man is the steward and protector of the flock. Veterinarians who provide euthanasia as a professional service are able to remain emotionally intact as long as they believe that they are doing the right thing for their patients.

Physicians wistfully express their desire for humane euthanasia for themselves if their own QoL declines to a worthless state or if it will help them avoid a slow, cruel, frustrating death. A large percentage of society readily convey similar desires for a peaceful and painless passing over the dreaded fate of being caught up in the gears of the mindless machinery of medicine.

One of this author's great mentors at UCLA Medical School feared that his advanced directive would not be carried out if he were taken by ambulance to the emergency room. When he knew that his aging heart was finally failing him, he went into his study to lay down on his favorite couch. He asked his wife to lovingly respect his wishes and not call the paramedics until his heart rate was well below 25 beats per minute. He specified that he did not want resuscitation attempts clearly in his DNR which he laid conspicuously upon his chest.

Mindless Machinery of Medicine

A survey of terminal cancer patients who elected salvage chemotherapy for recurrent disease found that a majority of the patients were under the unsubstantiated impression that chemotherapy could potentially cure them. (Weeks, et al.) It is well known that many patients in this situation endure chemotherapy related adverse events that compromises their quality of life or causes them to die badly in ICU's.

A survey of terminal lung cancer patients, who chose palliative care vs. standard care (further chemotherapy), found that the palliative care group lived 3 months longer and enjoyed a higher quality of life. In addition, patients and their family members were more satisfied than those who chose standard care. (Temel, et al.)

Veterinary medicine has evolved parallel with human medicine in its technical ability to resuscitate and maintain trauma patients, poison patients, organ failure patients, neurologic patients, etc. Decisions of whether or not to continue life support comes up much sooner with veterinary patients. This is because the pet owner is the financially responsible principle who must commit to pay in full for professional services rendered for their companion animal. Less than 3% of America's companion animals enjoy pet health insurance plans. Most of those plans have a $7-8,000 cap per illness or incident unless the pet owner purchased an extra cancer care policy. With facilities overhead, pay roll and urban expenses increasing, many pet owners find that medical care for a seriously ill companion animal can be costly. This feeling of expensiveness prevails despite the intrinsic value of services and cost of education and commitment of the veterinary profession. It is because financial responsibility rests solely with the pet owner that many elect euthanasia for their dying companion animals when faced with a poor prognosis for recovery or regaining an enjoyable QoL.

Delayed Referrals for Palliative Medicine and/or Hospice

Most physicians think that if they refer their patients for palliative care, it would exclude their "can do" standard medicine. Could it be that today's informed physicians, who eschew difficult conversations about bad news and death, still view palliative medicine in the same frame as hospice care?

Medicare and Medicaid might have caused this mindset when it was decided that life prolonging medical treatment for primary life limiting disease be excluded from hospice reimbursement. Is this misunderstanding, which remains pervasive in the medical profession, the real reason why physicians delay referrals? How can this outdated mindset be budged? Let this commentary make it well known that palliative medicine is not hospice although it may precede hospice.

There is no disagreement that American medicine is money driven and that the real needs of hospital patients, especially nursing home residents, exist in tension with regulatory goals. (The Hastings Center Guidelines) Are there rewards for physicians and facilities to blindly ignore patient needs, wishes and preferences and press on with their task-oriented, life at all cost philosophy of medicine? Why do physicians especially oncologists push onward with overtreatment? Why do physicians decline to refer patients out of their hemisphere of practice? What reimbursement motivators underlie the actual and rationalized truth in how physicians practice vs. what they would want for their own care? Why do physicians want less of the mindless machinery of medicine for themselves than they recommend for their patients?

One experienced counselor made this comment regarding her husband's end-of-life care in March of 2013. "*Doctors are not interested in the end game. Families are not offered hospice soon enough for comfort care. Doctors view hospice as giving up. Most Doctors want to keep the patient in the hospital as they try various medications to try to beat death back. Families who want hospice and do not want their dying family member's wishes disregarded must often have to fight for hospice care.*" Why is this mind set against accepting death as the last part of health care still the norm for so many physicians today when Vermont became the 4th state to pass aid in dying legislation and Quebec is leading the way in Canada?

PALLIATIVE CARE

Palliative Medicine can be delivered to patients regardless of an early or late stage diagnosis of a life limiting disease, regardless of the number of patient co morbidities or the need for other therapies. It can be delivered simultaneously with life-prolonging treatments or it can be delivered as the principle mode of care. The goals of palliative care are exclusively patient and family centered. This includes but is not limited to: preventing and relieving suffering while supporting the best QoL for patients and their families.

Palliative care is a philosophy of care delivered by interprofessional teams highly trained in communication to avoid cultural pitfalls. It expands standard medicine by embracing important end-of-life goals such as enhancing QoL for patient and family, optimizing function, helping with decision making and providing opportunities for personal growth. As of 2006, the American Board of Medical Specialties has recognized palliative medicine as a subspecialty of medicine, with an unprecedented ten primary parent boards. (Meier)

> "The hard question we face, then, is not how we can afford this system's expense. It is how we can build a health-care system that will actually help dying patients achieve what's most important to them at the end of their lives."
>
> Atul Gawande (2010)

Since 2000, the AVMA has recognized that palliative medicine and hospice care is beneficial for end-of-life companion animals in addition to euthanasia. Guidelines were developed that recommended practitioners who do not offer palliative medicine and hospice (Pawspice) services to refer clients to a colleague who offers this specialized end-of-life care. Both veterinary and human palliative medicine should ideally transition patients into hospice care when requested or when death is near.

Irresponsible and/or financially strapped pet owners relinquish their sick, old, incontinent, failing pets at animal shelters. Some are adopted by rescuers who might foster them or self-declared animal hospice care givers or sanctuary workers. Some are collected by hoarders who are mentally ill and blind to their suffering. Rescuers range from individual hobbyists to well run organizations, which employ various levels of veterinary supervision to almost none. A few eschew euthanasia and risk closure. Most seek donations to help their cause.

Disrespect of Advanced Directives

Physicians were trained to save lives by challenging death. Many view death as a defeat. "Not on my watch!" or "I don't discuss death with my patients." Doctors go into automatic mode when patients are wheeled into the emergency clinics which is the right thing to do for trauma patients and acutely sick persons. Many ethicists agree that "save life at all cost" may be the wrong approach for advanced age, frail people and for those with terminal disease who want to bypass and forego futile medicine via informed refusal.

For the oldest geriatrics, the admissions desk should conduct a deliberate quest for the person's wishes. A hospital wide policy should be in place to respect their advanced directives and DNR's. Sadly, in many scenarios, this is not the case. The emergency room doctors persuade family members to put their ailing, failing, frail parents on life support, intubations, tracheostomy tubes, feeding tubes, IV fluids, antibiotics, and a raft of other interventions and drugs, etc. Often, the patient wants to forego further futile medicine; however, they admit getting talked into it by their doctors or loved ones who want to avoid death at all cost.

Baby boomers are demanding that their advanced directives and DNR's be honored by physicians and family members or proxies. They want to be assured that today's medical system will support their right to die with dignity and according to their written preferences. Most people do not want to wind up unresponsive with gastric feeding tubes warehoused in the healthcare nursing system, which won't or can't address their desires due to disincentives resulting in an artificially protracted dreadful time that precedes their death.

Is the blatant disrespect of advanced directives and DNR's a philosophic, religious or ethical problem for emergency care physicians? Should these physicians hand the case over to a colleague who believes in honoring advanced directives? Is the common disrespect of DNR's simply the result of fear of litigation from relatives? Is it due to physician, "Not on my shift," avoidance of death? Could it be a money-driven scheme to keep the ICU wards full and keep the nursing care industry's beds full? If we examine the data on who wins by ignoring AD's and DNR's, the answers might be clearer.

Fear of Human Warehousing before Death

10,000 baby boomers turn 60 every day. Many are alone without immediate family members to be at their side when illness strikes. All fear deterioration at the end-of-life. They reject the system that puts declining old people out of sight and out of mind. They do not want to be one of those failing, frail, forlorn and forgotten bodies that fill the beds of nursing homes. Informed boomers want to forego the burden of cancer over treatment with one more chemotherapy agent. They want to refuse life-sustaining treatment whem facing multisystem failure. It is well known that some persons who feel disrespected, choose not to eat and die badly. How can caregivers ignore their fellow human being's cry for assistance to make a peaceful passage?

Modern society is all too aware that obesity is a chronic debilitating life limiting disease that chips away at the body with one minus after the other. Society knows that severely disabled, immobile and frail geriatric people are maintained in rest homes enduring further physical and mental decline. This is their fate despite their reluctance to move from their homes and giving up their pets. Their woes of poor quality of life and no reason for living are ignored.

An increasing percentage of modern society wants to exercise their right to a peaceful and painless passing vs. having to suffer humiliation and degradation as they decline toward death in a human warehouse. They don't want to slide down toward a non-functional and unresponsive state as their body joins the line-up for butts to clean and mouths to feed at end-of-life.

Oregon's Death With Dignity Act reported the top concerns of people who utilized their rights to physician assisted suicide in 2010. The top concerns were: 1) loss of autonomy (93.8%), 2) a decreasing ability to participate in activities that made life enjoyable (93.8%) and 3) loss of dignity (78.5%). (de Wachter) Surprisingly, pain was not one of the top patient concerns, which proves that adequate pain management is being addressed for most end-of-life patients and is appreciated in Oregon. The medical system forgets how important happiness is and how valued the ability to enjoy life is when considering one's quality of life.

AID-IN-DYING DRAFT

Rebecca Johnson, RN, Ph.D., FNAP, and the 2012-13 President of the International Association of Human Animal Interaction Organizations, gained experience in this arena while earning her doctorate at Iowa State University. She and her colleagues researched the intricacies and then drafted the Model Aid-in-Dying Act that could yield a potential policy/law. (Brandt, et al.) A hearing with Iowa state legislators concluded that the MD scope of practice, which viewed Aid-in-Dying as murder in 1989, blocked implementation. Johnson feels that this thinking or belief is still a major stumbling block in today's discussion. However, Oregon and Washington passed legislation allowing physician assisted suicide, Montana courts will not prosecute, Vermont passed legislation with aid in dying terminology, 6 other states have come very close in their voting for this measure and Quebec is pending.

Terminology can frame opponents with offensive names and skillfully loaded terms such as; "therapeutic homicide" or "death panels" or "culling grandma". Yet, the social ethic toward euthanasia is changing and views aid in dying as a much needed extension of health care. The conversation is highly motivated toward helping to solve a clearly unacceptable and sorry situation that has inadvertently and unjustly been created via modern technology.

One former rest home nurse said that her patients would often ask her to help them die because they were miserable and felt that their life was totally useless and not worth living. She always gave them her compassion and would hold a hand as she told them that it was not legal for her to help them die. She felt that her hands were tied behind her back during all those years on the job caring for hopeless unhappy people who did not want to be alive any more.

THE RELIGION ARGUMENT

Arguments based on religious fervor can cloud the real issues. It is very clear those who raise objections to death with dignity, terminal sedation, aid-in-dying and euthanasia are almost always based on religion or one's personal ethics or bias but not on science. Ideology inspires inflexibility and rigidly held myths and incorrect assumptions that defy and deny the complexity of people in contemporary society.

Most religious arguments from physicians and ethicists frame or declare certain behaviors as immoral or unethical for themselves, their colleagues and the entire human race. However, in reality these same behaviors may be routinely accepted in other cultures and other belief systems. An example of an imposed ideology for the universe is the condemnation of people eating horsemeat, despite the fact that 5 million horses were consumed by the human race in 2011.

All too often personal and/or religious viewpoints provoke a strong emotional clash of values causing barriers instead of negotiations. For instance, measures that make sense for an over populated or modern society, such as voluntary birth control or abortion, may be overtly opposed based upon the religious beliefs of a segment of that population, which are allowed to practice their faith. Yet, it is well known that some of the most outspoken political opponents will clandestinely seek these same measures for themselves and their families if needed.

Some opponents retaliate by adopting scare tactics. They might claim: the world will self destruct or that society will lose trust in the medical profession or vulnerable members of society would feel threatened or coerced to die. They claim potential harm (not proven harm) if the slippery slope toward physician assisted suicide, aid-in-dying or euthanasia became legalized.

Potential claims of harm were not problematic in the Netherlands where physician assisted suicide is not legal but permitted and not prosecuted for almost 2,000 people per year. (Van der Mass, et al.) Threats of harm and distrust for doctors haven't ruined the medical profession in Oregon or Washington or Switzerland or Belgium where physician assisted death is legal.

Many of the arguments against terminal sedation and physician assisted death will have difficulty holding ground in future ethical discussions, if they sincerely query, "What value is life if it has no quality? When is life not worth living? Why can't patient autonomy be respected at the edge of life?

Arguments from fixed beliefs or special interest groups are often stacked with: denial, misrepresentations, hyperbole, exaggeration, distortion, overstatement, understatement, smoke screens, veiled threats of potential harm. These techniques do not address the issues instead they are meant to blur the issues, block change and maintain status quo. Sadly, this unacceptable problem is growing and so is the moral obligation to do something about it.

USE OF DENIAL

The medical community claimed that there is not enough data on the number and nature of patient requests for medical suicide and euthanasia. (McMurray et al., 1992 AMA Council on Ethical and Judicial Affairs) This data might have been lacking because the questionnaires also asked physicians the number of requests that have been granted. It is well known that patient requests for assisted death have been honored for some time. (Wanzer, Federman, Adelstein) If the questionnaire omitted self-incriminating questions, the data might be more forthcoming from respondents. Rest home care givers can provide requested information for their population of patients.

Instead of denying that there is not enough data for the US medical and ethical community to operate with, a new open conversation could accumulate and use the available data and extrapolate. This technique is used scientifically with most surveys, polls and population studies. Care for death is ethical.

Since Oregon, Washington, Netherlands, Switzerland and Belgium have transparent documentation; their current data could be used and confidently extrapolated. Oregon reported loss of autonomy, inability to enjoy life and loss of dignity as the major reasons for requests for physician assisted death.

Open international conversations about the ethics of physician assisted suicide, aid-in-dying and euthanasia depend on trust and courtesy that both sides will be listened to and contemplated and will never be disparaged for holding opposing viewpoints. Truthful conversations are enlightening whereas framing, overt denial and confrontations are inflammatory and degrading. For instance, using words such as killing or homicide, is incorrect and inflammatory and denies that the patient has requested their death. Is it not the physician's role to minimize pain vs. preaching and proselytizing to avoid confronting death, which after all is part of life and undeniably unavoidable?

From Controversy to Consensus

The Society for Veterinary Medical Ethics uses the theme, *From Controversy to Consensus*, for its Plenary Sessions presented at the Annual AVMA Conventions. The great Leo Bustad, DVM, Ph.D., Dean, WSU School of Veterinary Medicine, is the renown father of the term, "human-animal bond". A collection of Bustad's thoughtful writings and speeches titled, *Compassion: Our Last Great Hope*, demonstrates his realization that as stewards of the animal kingdom, mankind has an innate compassion for animals. His leadership in forming the Delta Society (Pet Partners), the American Association of Human-Animal Bond Veterinarians and the International Association of Human-Animal Interaction Organizations, gave a springboard and credence to the changing social ethic to be kinder to the animals and the global environment that sustain mankind.

The question is. "Why should all physicians be forced to disallow their dying human patients the same innate compassion that society grants for animals?" If society considers it ethically detestable for a veterinarian or a farmer to refuse euthanasia for a miserably suffering animal, then the same principle should apply to change regulations that won't permit willing physicians to help suffering or miserable patients who ask for aid-in-dying.

New Language for Humane Human End of Life Care

Today's discussion needs new sensitive language to achieve change. Baby boomers have changed the world and they realize that they have more skin in the decisions that are being made about their geriatric future. They demand more respect for their AD's and DNR's and they want physician assisted suicide, aid-in-dying and compassionate euthanasia rather than waste away in rest homes deprived of pride and joy. Baby boomers are becoming pro active about healthy aging and how they want their end-of-life years to be spent.

The new language of assisted dying needs to adopt aesthetic words and euphemistic phrases such as: aid-in-dying, well death, quality death, helping terminal patients make their transition, peaceful passage, dignified departure, changing worlds (Barbara Myers), crossing over the rainbow bridge, leaving the body, peaceful and painless passing, compassionate release, gift of a good death, letting go, embracing the light, going home, final farewell, etc.

This new language needs to understand the religious fervor of those who oppose all forms of aid-in dying. Position statements by opponents should be honored as strong personal or religious beliefs, which are becoming more and more difficult to apply to all in today's society of multicultural and multi belief systems and modern technology. The new language can point out the damage that loaded terms create. Assisted dying advocates can deflate naysayers' dramatic inflammatory rhetoric. They can point out that selected phrases are emotionally loaded with the intent of suppressing independent thoughts and feelings with the intention for scaremongering. Is religiosity, indifference and denial ethically reprehensible when used to withhold aid in dying to alleviate pointless pain and or misery for end-of-life human patients?

Gentle Techniques for a Kind Passing

This commentary includes the ethics and rationale of using kind and gentle techniques for euthanasia of terminally ill companion animals and how these concepts may crossover to assist terminally ill humans. This author informs family members that euthanasia is a special service which we offer with reverence for life similar to a sacrament or a wake. We always provide a softly lighted room for our clients with blankets for the family to lay on the floor with their beloved dog. We bring flowers and candles to the room. We also encourage the family to bring their loved ones and household pets with them for this final goodbye to their beloved companion animal.

A heavy sedation is given IM, in the presence of the owner. This allows the patient to become totally pain free and to relax into slumber. This is the time that we help the family realize that their pet will lose consciousness in 5-10 minutes. We will leave the room to allow privacy but inform the family that the injection to follow is a strong barbiturate, which will cause their pet's heart to slow down and stop and the breathing to slow down and stop.

Our nursing staff will enter the room with me after a few minutes and place an IV butterfly catheter and deliver the euthanasia solution. During this time I have the client pet their dog's head and face and say goodbye.

If the patient is small, hypovolemic, hypotensive or dehydrated, we do not try to locate a vein to place a catheter. Instead, it is quite easy to locate the patient's heart and give the injection IC or if needed IP or into one of the kidneys or liver. We listen for a heartbeat and when there is none, the patient is pronounced deceased at that time. We often leave the room again so that the family can have privacy and hold a wake with their deceased pet. This is a special time which convinces the family that their pet will not wake up. We often come back into the room and sit on the floor with the family and read poetry from a special book, *Angel Pawprints* (an anthology of pet memorials), by Laurel Hunt. *Over the Rainbow Bridge*, (author unknown) is a favorite poem that describes eternal reunion and inspired Laurel to create this book.

The techniques described are gentle and compassionate and assures the family that their companion animal family member will have a peaceful and painless passing. (Villalobos) Occasionally, we euthanize a pet at exploratory.

All human health care workers need to allow themselves to absorb and consider how these concepts and techniques may crossover to assist the dying process for terminally ill people who request death with dignity. The aid-in-dying can be provided with carefully considered prescriptions which the patient can self administer. It would not be necessary for a physician to be present as his/her patient takes oral drugs prescribed under the careful scrutiny of physician assisted suicide, as patients and their families often prefer privacy for their passage. For end-of-life patients, unable to help themselves, palliative and terminal sedation are the most accepted techniques for aid-in-dying.

Despite many requests, veterinarians are not legally able to prescribe fatal drugs to their clients to administer to their companion animals for home euthanasia. Instead, a growing number of house call veterinarians who often use similar techniques described above, are filling the growing demand for in home euthanasia of America's beloved pets.

Veterinarians wear many hats. They serve as the one who may provide memorial keepsakes and makes arrangements for the pet's remains to be privately cremated, buried or rendered with the hospital's service provider.

Email tributes and eulogies are the new norm. Facebook and animal support web sites have become the place to memorialize a dearly beloved pet. Often the pet's family will make a donation to an organization that helps animals or does research to solve the disease that overcame their pet such as: Morris Animal Foundation at: www.morrisanimalfoundation.org, American

Humane Association at: www.aha.org, Association for Pet Loss and Bereavement at: www.aplb.org, Veterinary Cancer Society at: www.vcs.org and Animal Health Foundation at: www.animalhealthfoundation.org.

RETHINKING SUMMARY

The ethics and rationale of using kind and gentle techniques for euthanasia of terminally ill companion animals is presented in this commentary for consideration and crossover into human medicine. By 2030, one in five Americans will be older individuals at risk to endure social poverty from physical and psychosocial degeneration causing depression and loss of independence, mobility, memory, dignity, joy and desire to live. (Helfand)

As a veterinary oncologist, who has fought for remissions and quality of life, it brings great reprieve and relief knowing that most of my Pawspice patients will have a quality death. Providing emotional support and decision making tools such as the HHHHHMM QoL Scale for family members helps them make the final call for the gift of euthanasia. Some veterinarians might view this as a burdensome obligation; however, this oncologist views it as a professional privilege and an honor to alleviate pointless pain and suffering.

It is clinically obvious to this author that providing access to a quality death actually reduces the moral stress and distress of our oncology team while bringing great relief to the patient and their caring families. Today's social ethic frees veterinarians to kindly and compassionately usher their chronically ill and dying patients over the rainbow bridge, when the time is right. Modern society wants to be let off the torture rack of dying slowly or badly as well.

Imagine the day when AD's and DNR's become totally respected instead of creating ethical dilemmas for vulnerable family members and inflexible physicians to sabotage or compromise. Imagine if aid-in-dying becomes a personal choice for the chronically ill and aging human race at the end-of-life. Imagine having a role in the global health concern discussion and decision making that converges to offset the enormous magnitude of predictable human erosion, wastage, misery and cost. Imagine a world without forced end-of-life misery.

Imagine transforming end-of-life care from a fixed to a flexible decisional authority based on the individual's wishes. The courage and moral character it will take to change legislation to allow humane aid-in-dying for humanity would pledge willing physicians to recognize the patient's truth. This would create an end-of-life health care system that helps humans as humanely as veterinarians help their patients transition from a world of hurt.

RESOURCES

Aging Resources, Interprofessional Health Care: Working Together for Healthy Aging, National Academies of Practice, Spring Forum, April 5-6, 2013

American Association of Human-Animal Bond Veterinarians, www.aah-abv.org

Society for Veterinary Medical Ethics, www.svme.org

Pawspice, www.pawspice.org

REFERENCES

Animal Health Foundation: www.animalhealthfoundation.org

Brandt, C. et al., Model Aid-in-Dying Act. *Iowa Law Review, Oct., 75*(1), 1-125.

Bustad, L. H. (1990). *Compassion: Our Last Great Hope*, Delta Society Press, Renton, WA, 98057.

De Watcher, M. A. M. (1989). Active euthanasia in the Netherlands, *JAMA*, *262*, 3316-3319.

Helfand A. E. (2006). Aging and Chronic Diseases, Special Focus, from Public Health and Podiatric Medicine-Principles and Practice, 2nd Ed., American Public Health Association, Washington DC.

Hunt, L. (1998). *Angel Pawprints: Reflections on Loving and Losing a Cainine Companion*, Darrowby Press, Pasadena, CA, 91107.

Kaplan, L. (2012). So Easy to Love, So Hard to Lose, Jangen Press.

McMurray, et al. (1992). Decisions Near the End-of-life, AMA Council on Ethical and Judicial Affairs, *JAMA*, *267*(16)2229-2233, in Palliative Care, Eds., Meier, D. E., Isaacs, S. L., Hughes, R. G., Jossey-Bass, a Wiley Imprint, San Francisco, CA, 2010, 93-107.

Meier, D. E. (2010). The Development, Status and Future of Palliative Care, from Palliative Care: Transforming the Care of Serious Illness, Eds. Meier DE, Isaacs SL, Hughes RG. Jossey-Bass, a Wiley Imprint, San Francisco, CA, 3-76.

Morris Animal Foundation: www.morrisanimalfoundation.org

Myers B. 2012. The Magical Link: Love, Mystery and Other Secrets About the Bond Between People and Animals, Guardian Press.

Pierce, J., http://www.psychologytoday.com/experts/jessica-pierce-phd

Rollin, B. (2011). Euthanasia, Moral Stress, and Chronic Illness in Veterinary Medicine, VCNA, Vol. 41, No. 3, May, 651-659

Temel, J. S. (2010). Early Palliative Care for Patients with Metastatic Non–Small-Cell Lung Cancer New England, *Journal of Medicine*, *363*, 8, 8-19, 733-742.

The Hastings Center Guidelines for Decisions on Life-Sustaining Treatment and Care Near the End-of-life, Revised and Expanded Edition (2013). Section 4, Guidelines for Care Transitions, 89-103.

Van der Mass, P., van Delden, J. & Looman, C. (1991). Euthanasia and other medical decisions concerning end-of-life. *Lancet*, *338*, 669-674.

Villalobos, A. (1994). *Quality of Life Scale Helps Make Final Call*, VPN, Sept. Download most recent versions for dogs and cats at: www.pawspice.com

Villalobos, A. (2007). Canine and Feline Geriatric Oncology: Honoring the Human-Animal Bond, Blackwell Publishing.

Villalobos, A. (2007). *Euthanasia for the Geriatric Cancer Patient*, Ch.11, from Canine and Feline Geriatric Oncology: Honoring the Human-Animal Bond, Blackwell Publishing, 319-334.

Villalobos, A. (2011). Quality of Life Assessment Techniques, *VCNA*, Vol. *41*, No. 3, May, 519-530.

Wanzer, S. H, Federman, D. D, Adelstein, S. J., et al. (1989). The physician's responsibility toward hopelessly ill patients, New England *Journal of Medicine*, *320*, 844-849.

Weeks, J. C., et al. (2012). Patients'expectations about effects of chemotherapy for advanced cancer, *N Engl J Med*. October, *367*(17), 1616-25.

PAWSPICE & *"HHHHHHMM" QOL SCALE* SYNOPSIS

Alice Villalobos, DVM, DPNAP, developed "Pawspice", a program for quality of life (QoL), which starts when a companion animal is diagnosed with a life-limiting condition or disease. Pawspice embraces both palliative and kinder gentler forms of standard care to treat serious disease. It transitions to hospice [comfort care] as the patient approaches the final weeks, days or hours of life.

Pawspice protocols should not be considered synonymous with hospice which implies "giving up." Instead, Pawspice uses low toxicity standard care and immunonutrition to avoid adverse events and support QoL. Pawspice helps and counsels the family to simultaneously and consistently focus on pain and symptom management to improve QoL. Pawspice patients often gain longer survival times than patients treated with the standard "can do" approach.

The *HHHHHMM QoL Scale*'s scoring system 0-10 asks family members and veterinary teams to assess various criteria that compose basic QoL. Use the scale on an as needed basis [weekly, daily, hourly]. The acronym's five H's stand for: *H*urt, *H*unger, *H*ydration, *H*ygiene and *H*appiness and its two M's stand for *M*obility and *M*ore good days than bad days. This QoL scale also serves as a helpful decision making tool. It assists the V-Team and pet lovers as they struggle through the difficult and emotionally draining process of making the final call for the gift of euthanasia when it is needed to provide a peaceful and painless passing for a beloved pet.

A Feline QoL Scale may be downloaded at www.pawspice.com from the Quality of Life page.

In: End-of-Life Care
Editors: Maria Rossi and Luiz Ortiz
ISBN: 978-1-62808-555-6

Short Communication

CURRENT SITUATION AND CHALLENGES OF HOME END-OF-LIFE CARE FOR THE ELDERLY IN JAPAN: A QUALITATIVE RESEARCH FROM THE POINT OF VIEW OF NON-NURSE CARE MANAGERS

Yoshihisa Hirakawa, Takaya Kimata and Kazumasa Uemura
Nagoya University Hospital, Nagoya, Japan

ABSTRACT

Although a number of elderly people are opting to spend their last few years of life at home, elderly home end-of-life care has not yet gained popularity in Japan. In this short communication paper, we describe the current situation, and outline the challenges of home end-of-life care for the elderly in Japan using the KJ method as qualitative research tool.

INTRODUCTION

Due to the aging of the population, as well as the changing preferences of elderly patients and their families, a growing number of elderly people are opting to spend the last years of their life in a community setting such as their own home (Hirakawa Y, 2012). As a result, the community is expected to assume a growing responsibility in caring for the dying elderly. Improving the quality and quantity of palliative care provision at home has become an urgent priority in Japan.

Quality care management is one of the most important aspects of home end-of-life care for the elderly. In 2000, Japan introduced a special care management system under its public long-term care insurance which integrates care managers (Matsuda & Yamamoto, 2001; Tsutsui & Muramatsu, 2007). This system calls for care managers to make long-term or end-of-life care plans for the elderly, and for care providers to execute these plans. In addition, care managers are required to monitor and regularly assess the condition and level of satisfaction of the elderly and their families. Thus, along with family physicians and nurses, care managers play a key role in community care settings in Japan.

Family caregivers are often at a loss as to how to look after their loved ones, and need to rely on care managers. In 2009, we conducted a broad survey of 475 family caregivers of home bed-ridden elderly patients residing in Nagoya city to find out about the kind of information family caregivers seek and the way in which they generally obtain this information (Hirakawa et al., 2011). Our results indicated that family caregivers of elderly patients receive health information from their physician or from a care manager, despite the fact that care managers are not medical professionals.

Because care managers are involved in the care of home elderly patients from the early stages of nursing care to the end-of-life phase as total coordinators of home end-of-life care, they are knowledgeable about the situation and the challenges of home end-of-life care for the elderly from the view point of clients. However, very few studies have focused on this issue.

In this short communication paper, we will describe the current situation, and outline the challenges of home end-of-life care for the elderly in Japan using qualitative data from a focus group discussion among care managers in Nagoya City and the KJ method as qualitative research tool.

METHODS

Data Collection

We collected qualitative data through six-person discussions. First, six care managers took part in a ninety-minute discussion on home end-of-life care, jotting down all of their initial ideas and thoughts on the topic. Second, based upon these written notes, the participants spent another 90-minute session discussing the issue of home end-of-life care. According to the KJ method's empirical rule, discussions should be halted if they no longer yield new ideas or thoughts. Overall, study participants halted discussions on three occasions, as they felt they had covered the widest possible range of opinions and information at the time. Third, based upon these written notes, each participant drew up a complete list of all the ideas and thoughts generated during the discussions. Study participants were randomly recruited from facilities related to Nagoya University Hospital, considering a diverse range of characteristics such as age and workplace among the participants. Finally, the participants' ideas and thoughts were transferred onto 74 individual labels. All discussions were held in the end of 2012. Study participants were six non-nurse care managers from different home care support centers in Nagoya City (Table 1). The Japanese long-term care system provides care managers with official recognition as professionals whose primary responsibility is to oversee the coordination of care services and the formulation of care plans for elderly people. Licensed professionals such as nurses, physicians, social workers, and physical therapists, can be certified as 'care managers' provided they go through a special training program (Hirakawa Y, 2012).

Table 1. Participants' Characteristics

Participant	Age (year)	Sex	Career(years)
1	53	female	5
2	45	female	12
3	46	female	3
4	35	female	1
5	50	female	7
6	48	female	11

Abduction Using the KJ Method

We used the KJ method as a qualitative research tool. The concept and background of the method was explained elsewhere (http://mushin-kan.jp/;Raymond,1997). In summary, the KJ method (Kawakita's initials) was created in the 1960s by the Japanese ethnologist Jiro Kawakita. Aside from its application in ethnology studies (Yoshida et al., 2011), the KJ method is now widely employed in Japan as a tool for qualitative research and improvement of business operation. The method gathers raw, chaotic information from a specific setting and organizes it into manageable chunks of information. It is not based on fixed quantitative data and it does not aim to verify a hypothesis but rather to inspire a hypothesis (http://mushin-kan.jp/). The KJ method allows for information and ideas to be synthesized into a conceptual visual map using labels (Kawakita,1967; Raymond,1997; http://mushin-kan.jp/).

While this popular method is widely-used, there is only a very limited amount of literature explaining the standardized method procedure in detail. Therefore, both the author of the present study and a research assistant completed an eighteen-hour KJ method training course for researchers at Mushinkan KJ method training center in Kyoto (http://mushin-kan.jp/).

In addition to the six participants, the first author and his research assistant took part in the abduction. The exercise was performed in March 2013. As mentioned above, we compiled a total of 74 labels reflecting the thoughts and experiences of care managers on home end-of-life care provision.

The KJ method makes it possible to quickly and efficiently frame key concepts into labels. This procedure is called the multi-stage pick-up procedure. First, the author and the assistant picked up 32 out of 74 labels, using the following procedure: 1) decide on a target number of labels and select the number of labels to that target number, 2) read the labels silently and memorize them to get an overall impression, 3) mark the labels we wish to keep 4) in a second round of pick-up, mark the labels we wish to keep among the previously selected labels, 5) repeat this process until the resulting number of labels is close to the target number, 6) carefully select final labels. The target number of labels for the multi-stage pick-up procedure is generally required to be one-fifth of all labels to ensure the quality of the study.

Second, the author and the assistant organized the remaining 32 labels into groups using the following KJ method procedure (see Figure 1): 1) read the labels silently to grasp the entire image, 2) combine labels that share a strong similarity in substance, 3) set aside any label that stands apart ('loner'), 4) make a 'first-step nameplate' for each group of labels, 5) again, read the loner labels and first-step nameplate labels silently and combine labels that share a strong similarity in substance, 6) set aside any labels that stand apart, 7) after further reflection, make a 'second-step nameplate' for each group of labels. When grouping the labels, we endeavored not to follow standardized, stereotypical perceptions. Because the KJ method treats loner labels as separate groups, we ended up with nine groups (including three loner labels) following group organization.

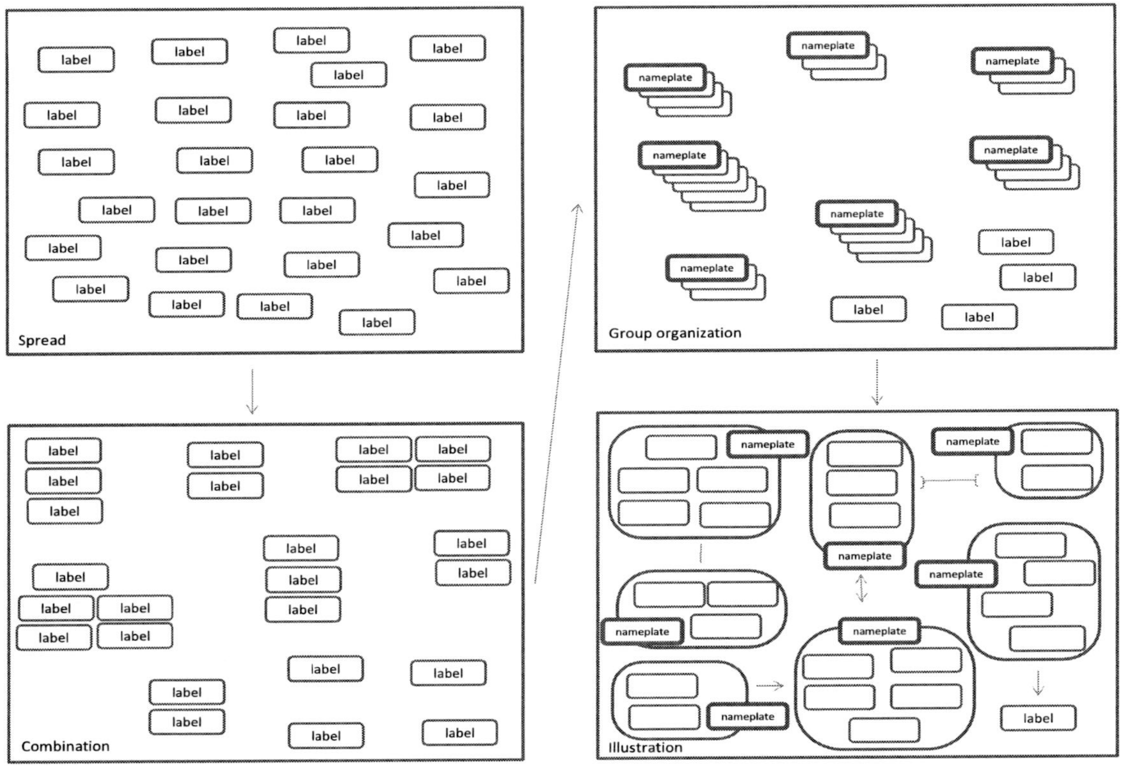

Figure1. KJ-method procedure.

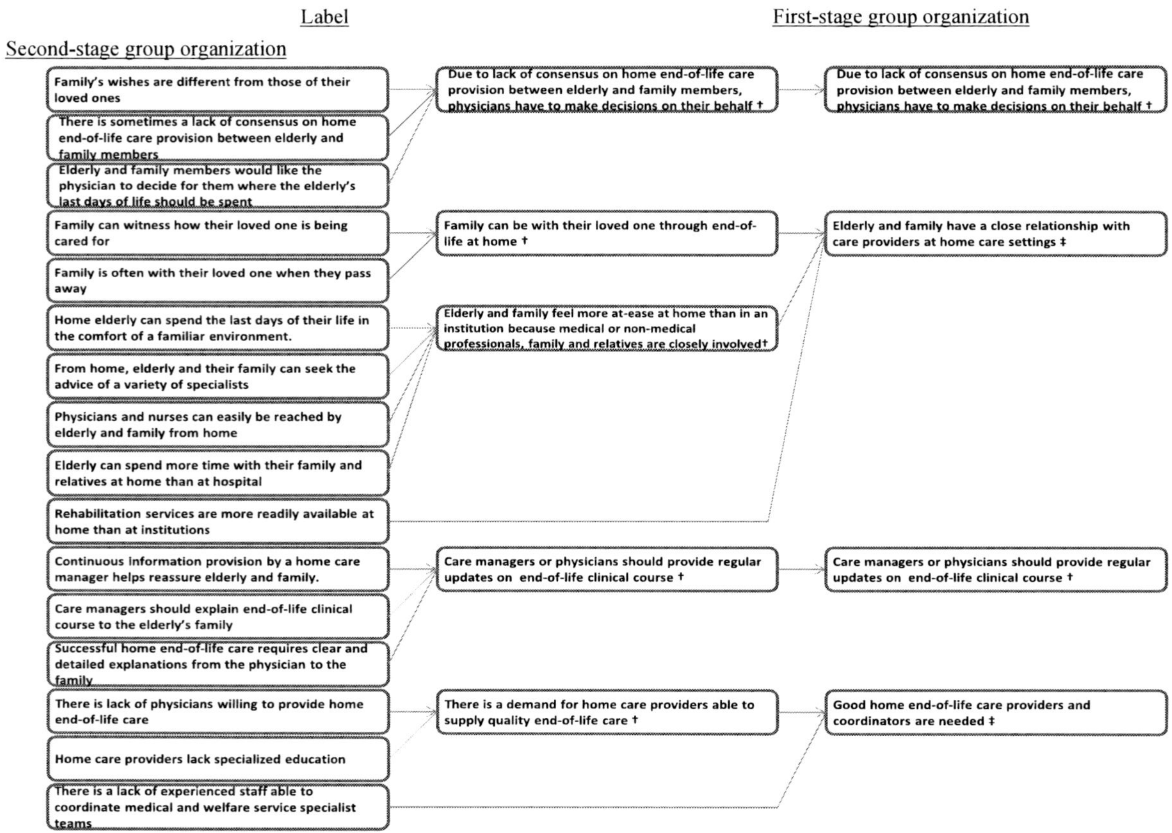
Label
First-stage group organization
Second-stage group organization
Family's wishes are different from those of their loved ones
There is sometimes a lack of consensus on home end-of-life care provision between elderly and family members
Elderly and family members would like the physician to decide for them where the elderly's last days of life should be spent
Family can witness how their loved one is being cared for
Family is often with their loved one when they pass away
Home elderly can spend the last days of their life in the comfort of a familiar environment.
From home, elderly and their family can seek the advice of a variety of specialists
Physicians and nurses can easily be reached by elderly and family from home
Elderly can spend more time with their family and relatives at home than at hospital
Rehabilitation services are more readily available at home than at institutions
Continuous Information provision by a home care manager helps reassure elderly and family.
Care managers should explain end-of-life clinical course to the elderly's family
Successful home end-of-life care requires clear and detailed explanations from the physician to the family
There is lack of physicians willing to provide home end-of-life care
Home care providers lack specialized education
There is a lack of experienced staff able to coordinate medical and welfare service specialist teams
Due to lack of consensus on home end-of-life care provision between elderly and family members, physicians have to make decisions on their behalf †
Family can be with their loved one through end-of-life at home †
Elderly and family feel more at-ease at home than in an institution because medical or non-medical professionals, family and relatives are closely involved†
Care managers or physicians should provide regular updates on end-of-life clinical course †
There is a demand for home care providers able to supply quality end-of-life care †
Due to lack of consensus on home end-of-life care provision between elderly and family members, physicians have to make decisions on their behalf †
Elderly and family have a close relationship with care providers at home care settings ‡
Care managers or physicians should provide regular updates on end-of-life clinical course †
Good home end-of-life care providers and coordinators are needed ‡

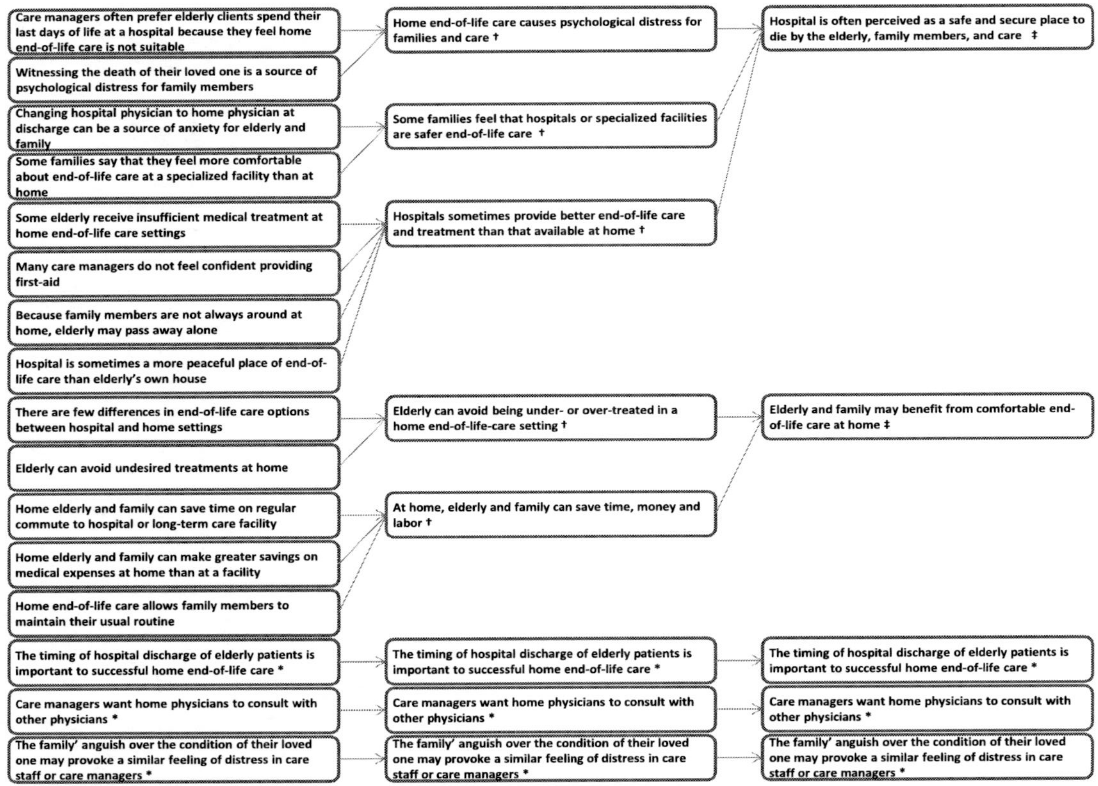

Figure 2. Flow chart of group organization.

Third, we arranged the groups with nameplates and the loner labels onto a large sheet of paper, paying attention to the inter-relationships between each group.

Finally, to confirm the clarity and cohesion of the group arrangements to study participants, we added a title that captured the overall message of the illustration and the relationships among the organized groups and loner labels.

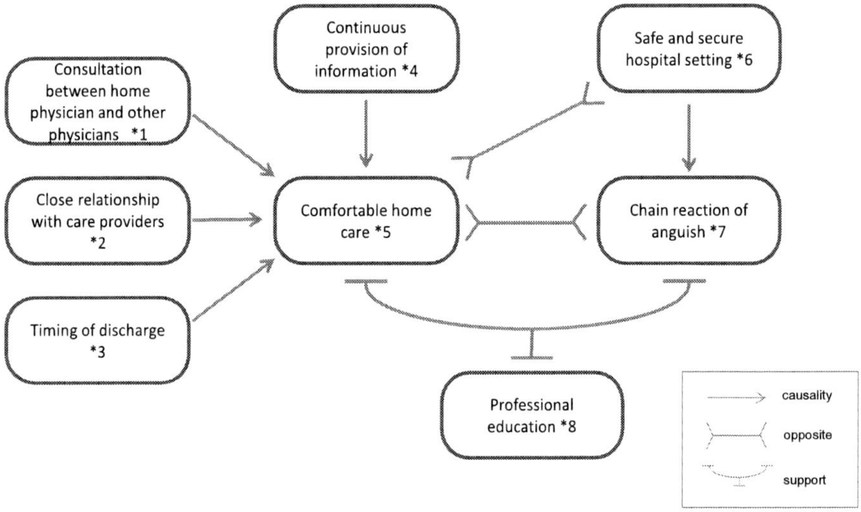

*1 Consultation between home physician and other physicians: The catchphrase of a label "Care managers want home physicians to consult with other physicians". *2 Close relationship with care providers: The catchphrase of 2nd-step nameplate "Elderly and family have a close relationship with care providers at home care settings" *3 Timing of discharge: The catchphrase of a label "The timing of hospital discharge of elderly patients is important to successful home end-of-life care". *4 Continuous provision of information: The catchphrase of 1st-step nameplate" Care managers or physicians should provide regular updates on end-of-life clinical course" *5 Comfortable home care: The catchphrase of 2nd-step nameplate "Elderly and family may benefit from comfortable end-of-life care at home". *6 Safe and secure hospital setting: The catchphrase of 2nd-step nameplate "Hospital is often perceived as a safe and secure setting to die by the elderly, family members, and care managers". *7 Chain reaction of anguish: The catchphrase of a label "Family' anguish over the condition of elderly may provoke a similar feeling of distress in care staff or care managers". *8 Professional education: The catchphrase of 2nd-step nameplate " Good home end-of-life care providers and coordinators are needed"

Figure 3. Illustrated figure of home end-of-life care is less practical, but less stressful than institutional end-of-life care.

This research was carried out with the consent of the Nagoya University School of Medicine Ethics Committee.

RESULTS

Figure 3 resulting from our group organization and illustration efforts was entitled "Home end-of-life care is less practical, but less stressful than institutional end-of-life care". As shown in Figure 2, the author and the assistant organized the 32 labels into groups using the KJ method procedure, and nine groups (including three loner labels) were extracted. Our results suggest that comprehensive training of end-of-life care staff is essential to sound and successful home end-of-life care for the elderly.

1. Group Organization

1) Due to a lack of consensus on home end-of-life care provision between elderly and family members, physicians often have to make decisions on their behalf.

   The label "Family's wishes are different from those of their loved ones" and the label "There is sometimes a lack of consensus on home end-of-life care provision between elderly and family members" suggest that it is difficult for elderly and family members to come to an agreement on home end-of-life care provision. Our results also suggest that "Elderly and family members would like the physician to decide for them where the elderly's last days of life should be spent".

2) Elderly and their family benefit from a close relationship with care providers in home care settings.

   This group includes the following labels: "Family can witness how their loved one is being cared for", "Family is often with their loved one when they pass away", and "From home, elderly and their family can seek the advice of a variety of specialists."

3) Care managers or physicians should provide regular updates on end-of-life clinical course.

   This group includes three labels: "Continuous information provision by a home care manager helps reassure elderly and family", "Care managers should explain end-of-life clinical course to the elderly patient's family," and "Successful home end-of-life care requires clear and detailed explanations from the physician to the family."

4) Skilled home end-of-life care providers and coordinators are needed.

   This group includes the labels: "There is a lack of physicians willing to provide home end-of-life care", "Home care providers lack specialized education", and "There is a lack of experienced staff able to coordinate medical and welfare service specialist teams".

5) Hospitals are often perceived as a safe and secure place to die by the elderly, family members, and care managers.

   First-step nameplates include: "Home end-of-life care causes psychological distress for families and care managers", "Some families feel that hospitals or specialized facilities are safer end-of-life care settings", and "Hospitals sometimes provide better end-of-life care and treatment than available at home". These nameplates suggest that hospitals are often perceived as a safer place to die by the elderly, family members, and care managers because they provide more adequate and timely medical care services.

6) Elderly patients and family members may benefit from comfortable end-of-life care at home.

   The first-step nameplates "Elderly can avoid being under- or over-treated in a home end-of-life-care setting" and "At home, elderly and family can save time, money and labor" suggest that end-of-life care at home is often perceived as more comfortable physically, psychologically or socially than at a hospital.

7) Loner labels

   The labels "The timing of hospital discharge of elderly patients is important to successful home end-of-life care", "Care managers want home physicians to consult with other physicians", and "The family's anguish over the condition of their loved one may provoke a similar feeling of distress in care staff or care managers" do not fall under any of the groups.

2. Illustration

The title of our illustrated figure is "Challenging yet comfortable home end-of-life care". Due to the immediate availability of medical care services in a hospital setting, many elderly and family members perceive hospitals as a safer place to die; they often wonder whether they should take their loved one to a hospital when they feel death is imminent. In addition, care managers or caring staff are often ill-prepared to face the challenges of caring for a dying elderly and handling death. The family's anxiety may intensify their feeling of confusion as to how to handle the impending death of the patient.

However, many elderly people and their family are now opting for home end-of-life care for a number of reasons, such as: 1) elderly can avoid being over- or under-treated at home, 2) elderly and family can save time, money and labor, and 3) elderly can spend their last days of life at home in a familiar setting. In addition, our results indicate that other factors suggest that home end-of-life care is an attractive, viable option: physicians' decisions on behalf of elderly and family, proper timing of hospital discharge to home, close relationship with care providers such as physician or nurse, continuous provision of end-of-life care information from physician or care manager, and consultation between home physician and other physicians.

Lastly, our illustration suggests that sound end-of-life care relies in great part on care managers who can adeptly face the demanding task of providing or coordinating home end-of-life care. Care managers are required to fully grasp the model produced by the present study results.

DISCUSSION

Due to a number of limitations to home end-of-life care provision including a shortage of qualified home care providers, a lack of involvement from 24-hour visiting nurse stations, and burden of family caregivers(Akiyama et al., 2007), elderly home end-of-life care has not yet gained popularity in Japan; in fact, although an increasing number of elderly people are now opting to spend their last few years of life at home, the proportion of elderly who do chose this option in Japan is still very low (18.3% in 1995, and 12.4% in 2009) (http://www.mhlw.go.jp/toukei/saikin/hw/jinkou/suii09/deth5.html). Although home end-of-life care offers many benefits, as our first-step nameplates suggest ("Elderly can avoid being under- or over-treated in a home end-of-life-care setting" and "At home, elderly and family can save time, money and labor"), providing quality home end-of-life care that adequately caters to the needs of Japanese elderly people remains a challenge. For example, as our results suggest, the fact that a family resides within easy access of a hospital often leads the family to forego their initial decision for a home death. For many, the anguish of personally witnessing the deteriorating state of their loved one may be so overwhelming that they may finally take the elderly to what they feel is a safer, more secure setting, the hospital. As our illustration suggests, there is a pressing demand for skilled home care providers or care managers capable of comforting family members facing the death of their loved ones at home.

Our results indicate that the guidance and support of a devoted physician throughout the decision-making process concerning home end-of-life care help promote successful home end-of-life care. Hattori et al. also stated in their paper that the will of elderly patients may easily change in view of the feelings of others (Hattori et al.,2005). Also, the Japan Geriatric Society suggested that Japan has developed a unique concept of life and death, and that Japanese elderly tend to avoid making decisions and are easily inclined to change their wishes, as represented by the patients' submissive attitude toward medical professionals (Japan Geriatric Society, 2012). Further studies are needed to expand on the present new knowledge regarding Japanese elderly patients' decision-making process at home end-of-life care settings.

The present study also indicates that the timing of hospital discharge of elderly patients is important to successful home end-of-life care. Fukui et al. previously revealed that the following two factors have an impact on place of death decision among home palliative care patients with advanced cancer: (i) pre-discharge health care support at hospital (e.g. early referral 8 days or more before discharge; clear explanation by hospital staff to patient and family regarding discharge in order to live and die at home), and (ii) post-discharge health care support after transfer to home care (e.g. signing a 24-h networking contract support insurance between primary physician and nurse as home palliative care team; primary nurse consultation with primary physician on three or more occasions during the first week after discharge) (Fukui et al., 2011). However, to our knowledge, very few studies have focused on the effect of place of death among non-cancer home elderly patients. Further studies based on our results are needed to further clarify this issue.

The merits of home end-of-life care, as our results reveal, are that "Home elderly can spend the last days of their life in the comfort of a familiar environment", and that "Elderly patients can spend more time with their family and relatives at home than at the hospital". These significant advantages of home end-of-life care have also been highlighted in literature. However, whether "Rehabilitation services are more readily available at home than at institutions" has not been confirmed, to our knowledge. Aside from home rehabilitation services available under Japan's long-term care insurance, elderly people can call upon the services of a number of home rehabilitation and massage professionals (Hirakawa Y et al., 2005). The fact that a wider range of rehabilitation options is available to home patients may have influenced our results, but this will need to be verified through additional studies.

Our results suggest that the regular provision of information by care managers or physicians helps reassure home end-of-life elderly patients and their family. Our results indicate that families usually feel equally reassured when a care manager instead of a physician provides updates and explanations on the patient's condition. Above all, meeting the information needs of family caregivers in a timely and appropriate manner is a key component of successful home end-of-life care. Our previous study exploring the information needs and sources of family caregivers of home elderly patients revealed that family caregivers were more likely to receive information from their care manager or physician than from any other source (Hirakawa Y et al.,2011). Our findings confirm these results further highlighting the need for care managers to be well-trained in home end-of-life care to be able to provide timely and useful information to the families.

Lastly, the loner label "Care managers want home physicians to consult with other physicians" suggests the importance of maintaining a clear line of communication between home physician and other physicians specializing in other fields so as to benefit from their professional advice and experience. To our knowledge, few reports have actually stressed the value of consultation between home physicians and physicians specializing in other clinical fields. Our results also suggest that there is a lack of trained family physicians qualified to provide high-quality primary care. In fact, the label "There is a lack of physicians willing to provide home end-of-life care" supports this hypothesis. In order to build a reliable home end-of-life care system in Japan, we need to provide quality primary care education and build a solid network of physicians specializing in different clinical fields.

CONCLUSION

The present qualitative study reveals that home end-of-life care can be a viable alternative to the hospital for many families, despite general opinion to the contrary. For home end-of-life care to be successful, the provision of timely information and high-quality primary care by skilled care managers and physicians is essential.

REFRENCES

Akiyama A, Numata K, & Mikami H.(2007) Factors influencing the death of the elderly at home in an institution specializing home medical care—Analysis of survey of the bereaved family—. *Nippon Ronen Igakkai Zasshi,* 44,740—746.

Fukui S, Fujita J, Tsujimura M, Sumikawa Y, Hayashi Y,& Fukui N.(2011) Late referrals to home palliative care service affecting death at home in advanced cancer patients in Japan: a nationwide survey. *AnnOncol,* 22(9),2113-2120.

Hirakawa Y, Kuzuya M, Enoki H, & Uemura K. (2011) Information needs and sources of family caregivers of home elderly patients. *Archives of Gerontology and Geriatrics,*52(1),202–205, ISSN 0167-4943.

Hattori A, Masuda Y, Fetters MD, Uemura K, Mogi N, Kuzuya M, & Iguchi A.(2005) A qualitative exploration of elderly patients' preferences for end-of-life care. *Japan Medical Association Journal*, 148(8),388-397, ISSN 1346-8650.

Hirakawa Y, Masuda Y, Kimata T, Uemura K, Kuzuya M,& Iguchi A.(2005) Effects of home massage rehabilitation therapy for the bed-ridden elderly: a pilot trial with a three-month follow-up. *Clinical Rehabilitation,* 19,20-27.

Hirakawa Y.(2012). *Palliative Care for the Elderly: A Japanese Perspective, Contemporary and Innovative Practice in Palliative Care,* Esther Chang and Amanda Johnson (Ed.), ISBN: 978-953-307-986-8, InTech, Available from: http://www.intechopen.com/articles/show/title/palliative-care-for-the-elderly-a-japanese-perspective.

Japan Geriatric Society (2012). [The Terminal Care of the Elderly- position statement from the Japan Geriatrics Society 2012], 04.08.2013, (in Japanese) Available from http://www.jpn-geriat-soc.or.jp/tachiba/jgs-tachiba2012.pdf.

Kawakita J.(1967) *Abduction* (Hassoho). Tokyo, Chukoshinsho. (in Japanese)

Matsuda S, & Yamamoto M.(2001). Long-term care insurance and integrated care for the aged in Japan. *International Journal of Integrated Care,* 1(1),1-11,ISSN 1568-4156.

Raymond S.(1997) The KJ Method: A Technique for Analyzing Data Derived from Japanese Ethnology. *Human Organization,* 56,233-237.

Tsutsui T, & Muramatsu N.(2007)Japan's Universal Long-Term Care System Reform of 2005: Containing Costs and Realizing a Vision. *Journal of the American Geriatric Society,* 55,1458–1463, ISSN 0002-8614

Yoshida I, Kobayashi T,& Teraoka S. (2011) A trial study on the use of a traditional folk song "Lam" for health education in Lao PDR. *Jpn J Health & Human Ecology,* 77,109-120 (in Japanese).

INDEX

C

D

E

F

G

H

I

J

K

L

M

N

O

P

Q

R

S

T

U

V

W

Y